The Cleveland Clinic Guide to

FIBROMYALGIA

The Cleveland Clinic Guide to

FIBROMYALGIA

WITHDRAWN

William S. Wilke, M.D.

KAPLAN)

PUBLISHING

New York

Published by Kaplan Publishing, a division of Kaplan, Inc.
1 Liberty Plaza, 24th Floor
New York, NY 10006

Library of Congress Cataloging-in-Publication Data
Wilke, William S., 1944-
The Cleveland Clinic guide to fibromyalgia / William S. Wilke.
    p. cm.
Includes bibliographical references and index.

ISBN 978-1-60714-489-2 (alk. paper)

1. Fibromyalgia--Popular works. I. Title. II. Title: Guide to fibromyalgia.

RC927.3.W525 2009

616.7'4--dc22

                                2009040984

Printed in the United States of America

10 9 8 7 6 5 4 3

ISBN: 978-1-60714-489-2

Kaplan Publishing books are available at special quantity discounts to use for sales promotions, employee premiums, or educational purposes. Please email our Special Sales Department to order or for more information at kaplanpublishing@kaplan.com, or write to Kaplan Publishing, 1 Liberty Plaza, 24th Floor, New York, NY 10006.

Contents

Introduction

Getting one's head around fibromyalgia syndrome (FMS)—what it is, how you know whether or not you have it, how it's treated, what the future holds—is not an easy task, for doctors or for patients.

Fibromyalgia is an elusive illness that affects between 6 million and 12 million people in the United States, or about 2 percent to 4 percent of the total population. The highest percentage of those diagnosed with fibromyalgia are women of childbearing age of all races; however, it does strike men, children, and women beyond their childbearing years as well.

While the symptoms of fibromyalgia syndrome haven't evidenced much change over time, in the past 40 years the definition of fibromyalgia and how it is diagnosed and treated have evolved significantly. Today you can find information about fibromyalgia almost everywhere. There are books, magazines, websites, and medical journal articles about it, and even television and radio programs. But some of these sources are conveying misconceptions. This book can help you sort through it all to find the facts.

We know that fibromyalgia is a physiological reaction (for some people) to stress. Stress can be external (job or family), environmental (workplace or world), or internal (emotions or physical illness). All types of stress can impair sleep and cause an abnormal production of certain chemicals that control how your nervous system perceives pain. There is also some evidence that genetics may play a part in how likely you are to develop fibromyalgia.

If you have fibromyalgia, you may have abnormally high levels of two chemicals in the spinal cord: substance P, which regulates how the spinal cord processes pain; and N-methyl-D-aspartate (NMDA), which stimulates the spinal cord as well as boosts production of substance P. That gives you a lower threshold for feeling pain. You may also have a lower threshold for tolerating light, odors, or noise. The resulting ultrasensitivity to pain and external stimuli is a hallmark of fibromyalgia.

The better you understand fibromyalgia, the more likely you are to develop effective strategies to ease your symptoms. It is my goal in this book to provide the tools you need to understand fibromyalgia, sort through the myths and misinformation, and conquer any feelings of helplessness.

I'll examine the history of how fibromyalgia came to be identified and look at the studies that have been done, and are being done, in the field, and why it's important for your doctor to screen for the causes of fibromyalgia even after diagnosis.

I'll explain how fibromyalgia is diagnosed and treated, and look at some startling connections between fibromyalgia and the physical world around us.

I'll give you and your family reliable coping strategies and trustworthy resources to continue your study of the disease beyond this book.

Whether you are newly diagnosed or have been contending with fibromyalgia for years, this book has something for you. Each chapter offers basic information about fibromyalgia for patients, their families, and caregivers. The sidebars and appendices include history and the results of key medical studies. And the case studies offer examples of people struggling to cope with fibromyalgia—and often succeeding.

There are many things that we don't know yet about fibromyalgia. But we do know that its signs and symptoms are not invented or imaginary. It's not a mental illness or a form of arthritis, although arthritis and many other illnesses or syndromes may coexist with it.

While we already know of many medications and lifestyle modifications that can ease symptoms of fibromyalgia and make everyday living more comfortable, extensive research continues to develop more, and more effective, strategies and treatments.

It is my hope that you will use this book as a guide and comfort as you pursue and undergo successful treatment.

Chapter 1

What Is Fibromyalgia?

Alice

It had been a bad year for Alice.

She turned forty in April. In and of itself, hitting the big 4-0 wasn't as awful as she expected. But the sagging economy led to the closing of an automotive outlet where her husband, Phil, had been the manager for seven years. Six months later, he remained unemployed, bringing in only a few dollars here and there from helping friends with car repairs. Money was getting tight. Really tight. So was the tension between the couple about whether Phil should go to work for his brother at one of his three car wash franchises.

Betsy, the oldest of their three girls, was a moody, argumentative 16-year-old, full of frustration that she dumped on her parents, especially Alice. Twins Erin

1

and Meg hadn't hit their teens yet, but between their interests in drama and band, it seemed that Alice did little but shuttle them to activities, work at her part-time job, and cook, clean, and nag.

Alice was always tired, and fell into bed every night feeling bone weary. Yet the minute she closed her eyes, the worry machine kicked in, and she'd still be awake two hours later. When she finally did fall asleep, she'd often wake up and toss and turn for what seemed like hours before dozing off again.

Most mornings, when the alarm went off at seven-thirty, Alice felt as tired as when she went to bed. Worse yet, for the past few months, the muscles and joints in her upper back and neck had been hurting big-time. She felt stiff and sore, especially in the morning.

One morning, after a nasty shouting match with Betsy about whether diet soda could be considered breakfast, Alice told Phil, "I don't know what's the matter with me. Every little thing bothers me. I'm shouting at Betsy, or the twins, or you, all the time. I can't sleep. Everything hurts. And I have to go to the bathroom practically every ten minutes. I don't know, I think my batteries are worn down, Phil."

"Not so run down that you can't go jogging." A bone of contention between them. The only time that Alice felt good anymore was when she was out for her daily run. She was up to an hour or more because the pain in her back and shoulders, even in her muscles, disappeared when she ran. Phil dropped more and more hints that maybe the pain and tiredness she felt the rest of the time were imaginary.

"If you feel so bad, why don't you go to the doctor and find out if anything's wrong?" he asked her.

The ifs didn't escape Alice's attention—did he think that the symptoms were all in her head?—but she made an appointment with Dr. Small, her primary-care doctor.

Dr. Small asked a lot of questions, especially about Alice's sleep patterns and when she felt the pain—and when she didn't. Then he performed the usual checkup. But this time, in addition to listening to her heart and taking her blood pressure, Dr. Small pressed on some of her muscles. When he applied pressure to the back of her neck and her shoulders, Alice winced and yelped, "That hurts!"

Dr. Small ordered a complete blood count and X-rays of Alice's chest, neck and lower back.

"Let's see what those tests turn up, Alice, and then we'll talk again."

Perhaps you recognize some of your symptoms in Alice's story.

Or you might be thinking, "I have the pain and the sleep problems, but nothing else sounds the same."

Fibromyalgia is a sneaky illness that can manifest in a number of different ways. But there is a core set of characteristic symptoms that lead doctors to suspect it.

There is always widespread pain that has existed over a period of months. There are no exceptions: fibromyalgia hurts, every day.

And there is always fatigue, almost always accompanied by sleep disturbances. We're not talking about feeling tired after a couple long days at work. We're talking about a continuing energy level so low that, like Alice, you feel your batteries have run down.

What makes fibromyalgia somewhat slippery to diagnose is that it doesn't necessarily include *or* exclude any or all of many other symptoms or syndromes, with the exception of pain and fatigue. (A syndrome isn't a formal disease per se, but rather a constellation of symptoms common to a group of patients.) Furthermore, no test, such as a blood test or X-ray, can definitively confirm a diagnosis.

Even more confusing, many fibromyalgia symptoms mirror those of other conditions, such as rheumatoid arthritis, chronic fatigue syndrome, depression, and migraine headaches. These conditions, and others, often coexist with fibromyalgia. This is why it's important for your doctor to look beyond the diagnosis of fibromyalgia to determine if you have other illnesses with overlapping or similar symptoms that also require treatment. Just because you have fibromyalgia doesn't mean that you can't have, for example, arthritis or lupus too.

Signs and Symptoms of Fibromyalgia

Your doctor diagnoses fibromyalgia by recognizing a specific pattern of signs and symptoms. If you have *all* of the following, you almost certainly have fibromyalgia:

- Chronic, diffuse, aching pain *at rest, and, especially, stiffness and pain in the morning*
- Disturbed sleep

- Chronic low energy
- Signs of stress such as worry, anxiety, or depression

We'll talk more about the steps doctors use to diagnose fibromyalgia in chapter 2. Now let's look in more detail at some of the symptoms and syndromes associated with fibromyalgia.

Do I Have Fibromyalgia?

Widespread Pain and Morning Stiffness. Widespread pain is always present with fibromyalgia, in soft tissues such as muscles, tendons, ligaments, and joints. Some people with fibromyalgia complain that they feel sore all over—the kind of soreness you might expect if you worked out at the fitness center for 6 hours instead of your 30 thirty minutes. Some say the pain is more like the all-over aching you get with the flu. Others describe muscle twitches or sensations such as burning, throbbing, or hot, stabbing pains. Most of your body hurts, although it may be particularly painful in your neck, shoulders, or spine. The pain may be worse in muscles you use over and over in repetitive motions. Morning stiffness and pain are frequent complaints among people diagnosed with fibromyalgia.

Fatigue and Sleep Disturbances. *Fatigue* is a vague word that can mean anything from temporary tiredness to chronic exhaustion or even sleeping too much during the day (hypersomnolence). For purposes of helping your doctor identify fibromyalgia symptoms, it's necessary to describe how you feel in detail. For example, low energy in fibromy-algia is characterized by the inability to sleep, feeling weak and listless, being unable to get started in the morning, and feeling as if your arms and legs are heavy. People with hyper-somnolence may take frequent naps and still feel tired. But tiredness from sleeping too much is a sign of a primary sleep disorder such as sleep apnea, not fibromyalgia.

Sleep disturbances play a big part in fatigue. Such conditions include insomnia, fitful or interrupted sleep at night, and sometimes even hypersomnolence. People with fibro-myalgia don't sleep well mainly because they do not get what is known as slow-wave sleep. We'll explore the physiology of sleep in chapter 2 and how it relates to fibromyalgia, but for now, it will suffice to note that brain chemistry and stress can influence good, restful sleep. Depression increases the production of corticotrophin releasing hormone (CPH), the stress hormone which acts directly on the brain to suppress slow wave sleep (SWS). And without restful sleep, fatigue can run rampant in the body.

Anxiety and Depression. Anxiety and depression are medical conditions with physiological causes that may be triggered by, or made worse by, stress. Fibromyalgia is a result of the body's reaction to stress, and therefore anxiety and/or depression almost always coexist with fibromyalgia. There are many disorders under the umbrellas of anxiety and depression, and we can't do justice to discussing these sometimes serious conditions here. However, some general characteristics and symptoms link them to fibromyalgia.

For example, most forms of anxiety include feelings of emotional or physical distress brought on by stress. Anxiety and worry go hand in hand. If you suffer from anxiety, you know how hard it is to relax and put aside your fears and worries. Most people with anxiety also experience one or more physical symptoms such as shortness of breath, muscle tension, dry mouth, backaches, headaches, and heart palpitations, as well as feelings of helplessness and irritability, and a lack of energy.

Depression involves the body, thoughts, and mood, and disrupts your ability to sleep, concentrate, or enjoy life. Depression, like anxiety, can include feelings of hopelessness and worry or sadness, and often brings about symptoms of fatigue, fitful sleep, and irritability.

Either of these conditions may be present without a diagnosis of fibromyalgia; however, fibromyalgia rarely is present without anxiety or depression.

Other Symptoms. Fibromyalgia sufferers often present with still other symptoms. Topping the list: chronic, recurrent tension or migraine headaches, which bedevil about 70 percent of men and women who seek treatment for fibromyalgia.

Another common feature is what we call central nervous system sensitization. I'll explain: your central nervous system, consisting of the brain and the spinal cord, is connected to the rest of the body by the peripheral nervous system. Just as the threshold for pain is lower when you have fibromyalgia, so is the threshold for sensitivity. Consequently, the world may seem too loud, too bright, even too smelly to people with fibromyalgia.

One way to understand sensitization is to imagine that all the nerves in your body and brain are overly sensitive, or, in medical jargon, up-regulated. Whatever you see, hear, or smell is magnified, as if the volume knob on the outside world is perpetually turned all the way up. A television commercial literally hurts your ears. Bright sunlight is unbearable. Your husband's aftershave, even though you know he just dabbed it on, smells like he dumped the whole bottle over his head.

Sensitization and another common symptom, cognitive impairment, are closely related. People with cognitive problems have trouble concentrating on things as simple as making a grocery list and balancing their checkbook. Sometimes this is referred to as "brain fog." These cognitive problems, and most other physical symptoms, are part and parcel of sensitization. Why?

Think about how we process information. Imagine, for example, that your son is sitting at the kitchen table reading you his essay on George Washington. You are making dinner. The television is on in the background, and you're half listening for the weather report. The buzzer goes off on the stove, but not before the potatoes boil over and smoke up the kitchen. The overhead fluorescent light imperceptibly flickers on and off.

How much of your son's report did you really hear? Your body and brain were busy filtering all the other noises, smells, and sounds in the room besides your son's voice. That's how it is for someone with fibromyalgia who experiences central nervous system sensitization: the nerves are up-regulated to the highest possible sensitivity all the time.

The excessive sensory information is overwhelming and distracting, making it very hard to concentrate.

Central nervous system sensitization in fibromyalgia can involve even the circulatory system. Arteries, the vessels that transport blood throughout the body, become abnormally tender, causing patients to hurt when they press against their chest, groin, and both sides of the neck.

Physical symptoms such as diarrhea and cramping, known as irritable bowel syndrome (IBS), the need to urinate frequently, and shortness of breath all are linked to the body's up-regulated state when fibromyalgia is present. The nerves in the bowel and the bladder become so highly stimulated that you feel the urge to go to the bathroom often.

The Forbidden Exes

Fibromyalgia is neither a diagnosis of exclusion nor an exclusive diagnosis—the two "forbidden exes."

What does that mean?

The diagnosis of fibromyalgia is not made by ruling out every conceivable cause of pain and fatigue; to do so, your doctor would have to perform potentially endless tests. Rather, fibromyalgia is recognized in a person with diffuse pain and fatigue who also has many of the other symptoms mentioned above. It is a diagnosis of recognition, *never* a diagnosis by exclusion. Therefore, a person with widespread pain at rest and poor sleep or fatigue very likely does have fibromyalgia. But it's also possible that he or she is suffering from rheumatoid arthritis, high blood pressure, migraine headache, or another condition.

Many people feel dizzy or light-headed when they stand up after lying down or sitting for any length of time, and sometimes when someone with fibromyalgia takes a hot shower, their muscles are relaxed and without pain, but they feel weak and a little shaky. This too is central sensitization at work.

Shared Symptoms

Back in the 1970s, when I first began practicing rheumatology and seeing patients with fibromyalgia, it struck me that although they came from all walks of life, they all described very similar symptoms—namely, the ones I've just described. And the similarities didn't stop there.

Almost to a person, they characterized their pain as constant even when they were resting. If they exercised or applied heat, the pain improved. But if they were exposed to the cold—being out in the snow, for example—the pain worsened. This got me thinking about the theory that fibromyalgia doesn't exist; that its symptoms are imaginary or side effects of depression. But these ideas don't hold up under logical scrutiny.

If the symptoms were imagined, wouldn't each person have a very different set of symptoms and clinical history? And although many patients I saw were depressed, not all were. The far more likely explanation was that their bodies all shared a common process that brought about their illness.

What to Do First

Perhaps you recognize yourself and your symptoms in this chapter. You have a stressful situation in your life and pain that won't quit even when you're sitting in a comfortable chair. You can't fall asleep, and on the rare nights that you *do* fall asleep, you wake up after just a few hours. And you have so little energy that your arms and legs feel like they have lead weights attached.

What should you do?

First and foremost, talk with your primary-care physician. Explain your symptoms thoroughly and honestly. Ask questions. If your doctor recommends laboratory tests or X-rays, ask what conditions he or she suspects you might have.

If your doctor doesn't mention fibromyalgia as a possibility and you feel strongly that your symptoms point to it, what should you do?

It's a fine line to walk. You don't want to undergo unnecessary procedures, yet you also don't want to refuse a test that might uncover a serious underlying disease and the culprit behind your symptoms. Before you undergo extensive tests, it is certainly your right to seek a second opinion with another doctor or a rheumatologist—a physician who specializes in diagnosing and treating painful and/or inflammatory disorders of the joints, muscles, and fibrous tissue such as tendons and ligaments.

And it is also certainly appropriate to ask your physician if your symptoms are consistent with a diagnosis of fibromyalgia. Do listen carefully and with an open mind to your doctor's reasons why he or she does, or doesn't, feel that fibromyalgia is a possible diagnosis in your case. Even more confusing, many fibromyalgia symptoms mirror those of other conditions, such as autoimmune disease like rheumatoid arthritis, systemic lupus erythematosis, or polymyagia rheumatica, as well as other diseases like parkinsonism or metabolic bone disease. Keep in mind that fibromyalgia mimics some serious conditions that you don't want to overlook.

A History Lesson

In 1904 the renowned British neurologist Sir William Gowers coined the term *fibrositis* (later to be renamed fibromyalgia) while writing an article on lumbago and other muscle pain syndromes.

In those days, the symptoms of fibrositis were considered to be a sign of hysteria, a common diagnosis that indicated a nervous disturbance. Gowers described the pain of fibrositis as equal on both the left and right sides of the body and recognized the importance of genetics when he wrote about the diverse occupations of his patients: "The patients have been elderly ladies of blameless habits and elderly abstemious clergymen, [and] members of conspicuously gouty families." The disease he referred to, gout, produces joint pain and inflammation, particularly in the big toe.

Gowers contended that the cause of fibrositis was hypersensitivity of the muscles supporting the spine. This suggested nerve involvement; a remarkably accurate conclusion, for we now know that the nerves controlling the muscles have become up-regulated. He also recognized that people with fibrositis were more sensitive to pain than they ought to be.

Gowers also speculated that tissue inflammation might cause the hypersensitivity; hence his coining the term *fibrositis*. (In the language of medicine, the word element *-itis* tells you that a health problem involves inflammation or an infection.) We now know this is not the case.

In 1974 Dr. Philip Kahler Hench, a California internist, took the formal definition of fibrositis a step further by proposing that primary fibrositis included aching, stiffness, tenderness, and pain in joints, muscles, and fibrous tissues in which there was no sign of another disease. He speculated that there was also a disorder called secondary fibrositis, which had the same symptoms but was caused by some other primary disease, such as rheumatism. The implication was that when the underlying ailment was treated, the symptoms of fibrositis would respond too. We now know that fibromyalgia can, and often does, coexist with other conditions and that treatment of *all* of them is necessary.

Three years later, Drs. Hugh Smythe and Harvey Moldofsky of the University of Toronto developed yet another definition for fibrositis. This one included widespread pain lasting more than three months, tenderness in certain body points, disturbed sleep, morning fatigue and stiffness, and the absence of any abnormal laboratory tests, such as blood or urine.

In a 1981 study, Peoria School of Medicine rheumatologist Dr. Muhammad Yunus and his research team compared the incidence of symptoms among 43 women and 7 men believed to have fibrositis and compared them with

50 healthy subjects. As you can see in table 1.1., the differences were pretty staggering:

Table 1.1—Symptoms in Fibromyalgia Patients Compared With Healthy Subjects

Symptom	Fibrositis Sufferers	Healthy Subjects
Generalized pain	98%	0%
Fatigue	92%	10%
Stiffness	84%	0%
Anxiety	70%	18%
Problems sleeping	56%	12%
Headaches	44%	16%
Irritable bowel syndrome	34%	8%
Swollen hands and/or feet	32%	6%
Numbness	26%	4%

Dr. Yunus also observed that cold weather, lack of exercise, anxiety, poor sleep, drinking alcohol, and exposure to air-conditioning made the symptoms of fibromyalgia worse. Conversely, a hot shower, massage, warm weather, and activity helped ease the disease's effects.

Yunus concluded that fibromyalgia produced widespread pain that lasted for at least three months. Another key feature: a minimum of five places in the body that felt tender when pressed. He also suggested that weather, temperature, activity, and stress or anxiety affected the severity of symptoms. In addition, the doctor perceptively noted no evidence of inflammation or infection, and so he changed the condition's name from fibrositis to fibromyalgia—*myalgia* meaning "painful muscle." It's been known as fibromyalgia ever since.

Chapter 2

Diagnosing Fibromyalgia

Alice

When Alice returned to see Dr. Small two weeks later, he seemed puzzled.

"Alice," he said, "you have a lot of symptoms that suggest fibromyalgia. The fatigue, the pain, the sleep issues, and irritability. Your blood test results were all within the normal range, and so were the X-rays of your chest, neck, and lower back."

Alice was relieved. She'd been half afraid that Dr. Small, like her husband, would say her symptoms were imaginary.

"I'm glad my test results are good," said Alice. "What is fibromyalgia? I've heard of it, but ..."

"Fibromyalgia is an illness or clinical syndrome that is characterized by chronic widespread pain, fatigue,

sleep disturbance, and muscle tenderness—all symptoms you exhibit. But when I examined you, I found only four areas of tenderness, which we refer to as tender points. Of the eighteen we test, you should have tenderness in at least eleven of them in order to make a diagnosis of fibromyalgia."

Alice's spirits sagged. If she didn't have fibromyalgia, what did she have?

"So what do you think is wrong with me, then? Is there something else you think it might be? Or do you think this is all in my head?"

"I do not think it is your imagination, Alice. If I did, I'd refer you to a good psychologist. But there aren't any tests or biopsies that will conclusively confirm fibromyalgia."

Alice laughed. Just hearing Dr. Small say that he didn't think she was making up her symptoms came as a big relief.

"So what's next, then?"

"Next is that I want you to see a rheumatologist. There are other specialists I could suggest to rule out some possibilities, but a rheumatologist seems like the best and most logical place for you to start. Diagnosing fibromyalgia is primarily a process of identifying the characteristics of your pain and distinguishing it from either a rheumatic condition or another, sometimes serious, disease."

Dr. Small explained that the rheumatologist might refer her to still other doctors for tests, such as an endocrinologist to screen for thyroid or adrenal gland dysfunction or a neurologist to investigate the possibility of a primary muscle disease.

"The thing is," he continued, "you may have more than one condition at work here, Alice, and the rheumatologist will want to check you out thoroughly, although once the diagnosis is made, you may be referred back to me for ongoing care and treatment."

Alice wasn't sure she liked the idea of seeing someone besides Dr. Small, but she reluctantly agreed to set up an appointment at the Cleveland Clinic's Department of Rheumatic and Immunologic Diseases.

Alice's visit to the Cleveland Clinic would be the beginning of long, sometimes frustrating but ultimately rewarding journey back to feeling better and assuming control of her health and her life.

Dr. Small was an astute physician. He recognized the symptoms of fibromyalgia, understood that it can be complex to diagnose, and sent Alice to a rheumatologist for a thorough workup.

Even more importantly, Dr. Small believed that her symptoms were real and that fibromyalgia is a real illness. All too often, that is not the case, and many people suffer needlessly before finding appropriate medical help. Let's take a look at some of the ways that physicians arrive at a diagnosis of fibromyalgia.

Figure 2.1—*Tender Points*

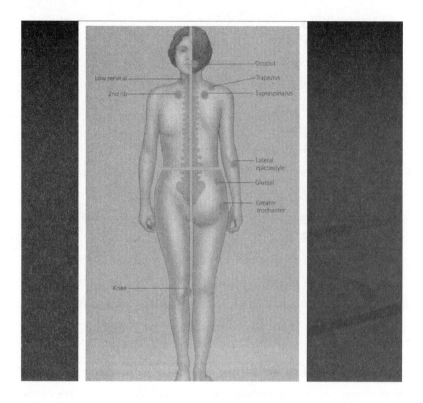

Tender Points

Drs. Smythe and Moldofsky developed their own diagnostic criteria for fibrositis in 1977. It included, among other features, tenderness or pain at 12 of the 14 sites that they identified and were the first to call tender points. Not long afterward, Dr. Yunus reduced the number of tender points necessary to warrant a diagnosis to 5.

To accurately measure the level of pain at tender points, doctors use an instrument called a dolorimeter. The spring-loaded tube-shaped device is held against the area in question while the pressure against the body is slowly increased. People with fibromyalgia will often experience pain at tender points with just moderate pressure, or less than 4 kilograms. In contrast, people without fibromyalgia won't notice any discomfort until the pressure is at least 6 kilograms.

As it turns out, for someone with normal blood pressure, 4 kilograms is about the pressure it takes to change the color of the nail bed on a person's finger. Doctors discovered that they could press a tender point with their thumbs and obtain a reasonably accurate reading of the pressure applied without using a dolorimeter.

In 1990, after much discussion, the American College of Rheumatology (ACR) established two mandatory criteria for diagnosing fibromyalgia: the presence of widespread pain for at least three months, and tenderness in at least 11 of 18 tender points. The tender-point standard had some loopholes, however. For example, someone might have pain in 12 tender points, but only above the waist. That would strongly suggest something other than fibromyalgia is going on, because fibromyalgia involves the entire body.

Since 1990, other criteria, such as the Manchester criteria developed in the United Kingdom, have redefined chronic widespread pain and deemphasized counting tender points when diagnosing fibromyalgia. One important study, the 1997 London Fibromyalgia Epidemiology Study Screening Questionnaire (LFESSQ), led to the first tool to screen for fatigue as well as pain.

In current practice, doctors rely less on tender points and more on symptoms. Today the Symptom Intensity Scale (figure 2.2) can be used to make the diagnosis of fibromyalgia without the need for examination. The SIS asks patients whether they have had pain in any of 19 areas of the body and to rate their fatigue on a scale of 1 to 10. You may well have fibromyalgia if (1) you have pain all over, (2) you check "yes" to pain in any 8 areas on the SIS, and (3) you have a fatigue score of greater than 6, It's important for your doctor to then be sure that you do not have other diseases which, although unrelated, can also be present. The SIS may also be

Figure 2.2—*Symptom Intensity Scale*

Symptom Intensity Scale

Please indicate any areas of pain in the past 7 days

AREAS	YES	NO	AREAS	YES	NO
Jaw (left)	____	____	Upper arm (left)	____	____
Jaw (right)	____	____	Upper arm (right)	____	____
Chest	____	____	Upper back	____	____
Abdomen	____	____	Hip (left)	____	____
Forearm (left)	____	____	Hip (right)	____	____
Forearm (right)	____	____	Shoulder (left)	____	____
Upper leg (left)	____	____	Shoulder (right)	____	____
Upper leg (right)	____	____	Neck	____	____
Lower leg (left)	____	____	Lower back	____	____
Lower leg (right)	____	____			

Total number of painful areas: ____
(this is the Regional Pain Scale score)

Please indicate your current level of fatigue

No fatigue |——————————————————————————————————| Very fatigued

(Measure the position of the patient's response in centimeters from the left end of this 10-cm line. This is the fatigue visual analogue scale score.)

Survey Criteria for fibromyalgia syndrome:
Regional Pain Scale score of 8 or higher and fatigue visual analogue scale score 6 cm or higher[a]

Symptom Intensity Scale score =
[Fatigue visual analogue scale + (Regional Pain Scale score / 2)]/2[b]

---

[a]A score of 5.0 cm or higher on the fatigue visual analogue scale is probably consistent with a diagnosis of fibromyalgia syndrome.
[b]A score ≥ 5.75 is diagnostic and differentiates fibromyalgia syndrome from other rheumatic conditions.

used to measure the severity of fibromyalgia, which, if you think about it, also measures the severity of distress.

Tender points are still important, although it's no longer necessary to have a certain number for a diagnosis of fibromyalgia. They're helpful in determining the severity of fibromyalgia and quantifying underlying stress factors such as depression and anxiety.

What to Expect

Because fibromyalgia shares symptoms with many other conditions and cannot be confirmed by laboratory or other tests, it can easily be overlooked initially and go untreated.

Some conditions that commonly coexist with fibromyalgia are anxiety, irritable bowel syndrome, depression, sleep apnea, and chronic migraine or tension headaches. Symptoms of fibromyalgia may also be shared with serious diseases such as hypothyroidism or polymyalgia rheumatica.

Any of the above conditions or diseases must be diagnosed and treated, *as must fibromyalgia.* In far too many cases, however, once an illness or disease that can be diagnosed by laboratory tests or other procedures is confirmed, the search for other conditions stops. Unfortunately for many patients, the pain, tenderness, and unrelenting fatigue do not. The good news is that the symptoms of fibromyalgia are becoming better known, both among patients and physicians, which often results in a timelier and more accurate diagnosis of not only fibromyalgia but coexisting conditions as well.

There is no typical scenario to illustrate how someone comes to be diagnosed with fibromyalgia. Sometimes your primary-care doctor, like Dr. Small, will refer you directly to a rheumatologist to handle your diagnosis and treatment. In other cases, your primary-care doctor may not feel a referral to a specialist is necessary.

The key element is that you find a doctor, whether it's your primary-care doctor or a specialist, who knows what fibromyalgia is, how to diagnose it, and how to treat it— and that *you* become well informed about the illness as well. Reading this book is a good start.

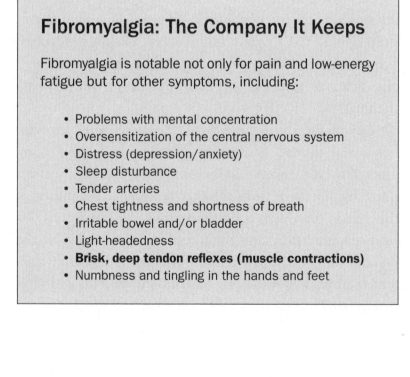

Fibromyalgia: The Company It Keeps

Fibromyalgia is notable not only for pain and low-energy fatigue but for other symptoms, including:

- Problems with mental concentration
- Oversensitization of the central nervous system
- Distress (depression/anxiety)
- Sleep disturbance
- Tender arteries
- Chest tightness and shortness of breath
- Irritable bowel and/or bladder
- Light-headedness
- **Brisk, deep tendon reflexes (muscle contractions)**
- Numbness and tingling in the hands and feet

• • • *Fast Fact* • • •

There are no definitive laboratory or X-ray tests for fibromyalgia. We base the diagnosis on a thorough medical exam, including a detailed patient history, and an evaluation of your symptoms. If something in your history or exam leads your doctor to suspect you may have something going on in addition to fibromyalgia, he or she may recommend laboratory or other diagnostic tests to confirm or rule out a coexisting condition.

In some cases, tests are done to rule out other conditions *before* fibromyalgia is confirmed. This can be time consuming, expensive, even painful—and always unnecessary, unless symptoms suggest the presence of another illness or disease in addition to fibromyalgia. (See pages 56–57 on tests not to have.)

Although self-diagnosis carries some risks, and remembering that fibromyalgia is not an exclusive diagnosis meant to explain every symptom you might have, you can obtain a good estimate of whether or not you have fibromyalgia by simply completing a Symptom Intensity Scale. A score of 5 or higher is a good indication that you have fibromyalgia.

• • •

A Visit to Dr. Wilke

On any given day, I walk into an examining room and meet a patient with an account similar to the one that follows, the story of a middle-aged woman I'll call Elaine, who has already been to a round-robin of specialists in order to explain the cause of her unrelenting pain and low energy.

Before even meeting Elaine, I knew from a quick review of her file and her previous visits to other doctors that she and her referring internist were desperate to discover why she was having so many unexplainable symptoms, including pain in her back and neck. According to Elaine's history, she went to her primary-care doctor about five months ago with complaints of neck and back pain and fatigue. Her doctor ordered some routine tests, such as a complete blood count and an X-ray of her back and neck. Not surprisingly, Elaine's doctor, like Alice's, found nothing in the results to explain the pain and low energy.

Elaine saw several other doctors, including an endocrinologist, a neurologist, and a back specialist. None found any underlying disease, but the back specialist told Elaine that she might have fibromyalgia, which led her to consult with me.

Her first words when I walked into the examining room were, "Is this all in my head? You're my last hope!"

We talked about Elaine's medical history and lifestyle. She'd had some medical problems over her 48 years, but nothing that led me to suspect they might contribute to her pain. She said she was happy with her job as a third-grade teacher until three years ago, when a new principal was hired. Elaine had loved teaching. The new principal changed all that.

"He can be so negative," Elaine explained. "We just don't see eye to eye on how to educate children, and it's really dragging me down."

The tension had escalated to the point that Elaine was utterly exhausted by the time she got home from work.

"I just have no energy anymore," she complained. Despite being tired all the time, she had trouble falling asleep and often woke up during the night. She said that the pain in her back and neck started around the time when she quit going to exercise class.

"I hurt all over, all the time," Elaine said. "It doesn't matter if I'm sitting or standing or walking around the grocery store. I hurt. And I can hardly remember my name, let alone what's on my grocery list, which isn't like me."

So far, everything Elaine told me sounded like fibromyalgia. She had constant pain for more than three months. She described the kind of low-energy fatigue typical of fibromyalgia. She had lots of stress in her life, and she had sleep difficulties. And according to her records, all the tests that she'd undergone looking for conditions or diseases that might cause such symptoms came back negative.

"Let me ask you some questions, Elaine."

"Sure, go ahead!"

"Have you noticed that bright lights, loud noises, or strong smells bother you more than they did in the past?"

"Noise for sure." she said. "I'm always telling my husband, Fred, to turn the television down. And maybe smells, too, now that you mention it."

"Any sore throat symptoms?" Tender carotid arteries are often perceived as a sore throat.

She shook her head but said she did have a lot of tenderness when she swallowed.

"And I'm getting more headaches these days," she added.

So far everything fit. I asked her if she'd had any stomach problems or difficulty with her bowels.

"Yes, I get cramps a lot and constipated sometimes. And I always feel like I have to urinate."

"Like you're bladder's too sensitive?"

She nodded.

"If you sit for a while and suddenly stand, do you ever get dizzy or light-headed?"

Elaine rubbed her hands together nervously. "Yes. That's been happening in my classroom, but I didn't want to tell anyone. I thought I might be having little strokes. I was so scared. And sometimes I get tingling in my hands and feet."

Then I asked the clincher question:

"When you take a hot shower, does it soothe your muscles but make you feel weak afterward?"

Elaine stared at me. "Yes. How did you know that?"

I explained that Elaine's history and test results led me to believe that the back specialist was right and fibromyalgia was at the root of her troubles. Her answers to my questions helped assure me that I was on the right track. Nevertheless, there was still additional ground to cover, such as helping Elaine understand fibromyalgia.

"How did I get this?" she wanted to know.

Good question.

What Are the Roles of Stress and Sleep in Contributing to Fibromyalgia?

"Let's go back to the hiring of that new principal," I said to Elaine.

I could see her body tense.

"Okay."

"He's added stress to your life, right?

"Oh, yeah."

"Here's what happens when you have an onset of stress in your life: stress interferes with sleep. If we don't get plenty of good, deep sleep, our bodies don't make certain brain chemicals that control how our nerves respond, or fire, in response to a stimulus. One of your first symptoms was interrupted sleep."

Elaine nodded.

"Did the rest of the symptoms seem to develop after the problems with sleeping began?"

"I guess."

She agreed that she wasn't very happy these days—and the symptoms she'd been having and the lack of a diagnosis only made her feel worse. "To tell you the truth, I'm a little depressed."

I explained how depression, too, can disturb good sleep.

When I asked her if anyone else in her family experienced problems with sleep and stress, she replied, "Yes. My mom. She's always been a worrier and wanders around the house half the night."

"These sorts of symptoms do tend to run in families." I sat back and folded my arms. "So, Elaine. After all this information I've dumped on you, what do *you* think is wrong with you?"

"I'm too sensitive?" she answered, with a hint of a smile.

"Yes," I said. "That's it exactly. Fibromyalgia is a matter of sensitivity."

What Diagnostic Tests Will I Undergo?

Elaine was relieved to learn there was a name for what she'd been experiencing—that it wasn't "head problems," as her husband had once called her symptoms.

I explained to Elaine that even though I had no doubt fibromyalgia was the cause of her symptoms, we still needed to talk about some other possibilities to make sure we didn't overlook a coexisting problem.

Some of the information was already in her medical file, but I, like most doctors, prefer to talk directly to the patient and perform a physical exam. It's easy to misinterpret another doctor's comments, and her condition might have changed, even in just a few weeks' time. It's always better *not* to assume anything when confirming a patient's diagnosis.

• • • Fast Fact • • •

General medical studies show how important it is for your physician to use all three tools—patient history, physical exam, and laboratory tests—to reach any definitive diagnosis. One study established that while doctors are able to predict a correct diagnosis about 76 percent of the time after taking a medical history, the percentage of confirmed diagnoses goes up to 89 percent after the physical exam is completed. And it is only after laboratory testing is done that the final 11 percent of cases are diagnosed.

Because no blood tests or X-rays can be used to diagnose fibromyalgia, the history becomes even more important. Tools like the SIS are invaluable. The physical examination is also crucial, especially to detect tenderness indicative of fibromyalgia, and any signs which might indicate simultaneous unrelated conditions If laboratory tests and/or X-rays are ordered, it's strictly to rule out other disorders that bring about similar symptoms.

• • •

Here are some of the areas I covered with Elaine in discussing her personal medical history:

- The possibility of an autoimmune disease such as rheumatoid arthritis or lupus erythematosus.
- A past history of anemia (a deficiency of red blood cells), or abnormal white blood cell or platelet counts
- Inflammatory muscle diseases such as polymyagisis
- Dry eyes or the need to use eye drops as occurs in Sjögren's syndrome
- Past surgeries or blood transfusions
- Sleep apnea

I also conducted a physical exam during which I checked for narrowed carotid arteries, swollen joints, and tenderness. (The carotids are a pair of vital blood vessels that supply the head. Narrowness may indicate atherosclerosis, or hardening of the arteries, a potential risk factor for dementia and stroke.) The tenderness was widespread, as I would have expected given the sensitivity of her nerves.

In order to determine the severity of Elaine's illness, I used several questionnaires, or scales, including:

- Fibromyalgia Impact Questionnaire—The FIQ consists of 10 questions designed to evaluate the quality of life and the degree to which fibromyalgia interrupts daily activities. The first question is composed of 11 items related to your ability to perform large-muscle tasks and is often referred to as the Fibromyalgia Impact Questionnaire Disability Index (FIQ-DI). For example, it asks if fibromyalgia prevents you from going shopping or preparing meals (0) always, (1) most of the time, (2) occasionally, or (3) never. The FIQ-DI predicts, better than any other tool or test, a patient's improvement or nonimprovement. The next 3 scales measure the impact of fibromyalgia on your work and activity, and the final 6 measure the severity of the primary symptoms. When I give the FIQ, I add a 7th scale, which measures sleep quality. This flexibility makes the FIQ a very useful and necessary tool to determine the severity of specific symptoms and their effects on the quality of life in patients with fibromyalgia.

- Symptom Intensity Scale—The SIS, mentioned previously, facilitates diagnosis and measures the severity of fibromyalgia.

- Epworth Sleepiness Scale—I use the ESS instead of a fatigue scale alone. Fatigue scales typically measure only whether a patient has low energy and/or hypersomnolence, whereas the Epworth Sleepiness Scale identifies what's causing the symptoms, such as sleep apnea, narcolepsy, or restless legs syndrome, I can then refer patients who are identified to have these types of disorders to one of my colleagues in sleep medicine.

• Depression Scales—The degree of a patient's depression is a good indicator of the severity of fibromyalgia. One of the Fibromyalgia Impact Questionnaire scales measures mood, as do other questionnaires such as the Beck Depression Index (BDI) or parts of the Arthritis Impact Activity Scale. In addition to one of those scales, I have all my patients complete the Mood Disorders Questionnaire (MDQ), which asks 13 yes or no questions to screen for a history of impulsive (hypomanic) or very impulsive (manic) behavior. (Sample question: "Have you ever felt so good that other people thought you were not your normal self?")

Other questionnaires can be used besides the ones mentioned here, including measures of helplessness and anxiety, and instruments such as pain drawings, which may determine how severe the symptoms and central sensitization are in a fibromyalgia patient. A pain drawing is just what it sounds like: two simple line drawings of the human form, front and back, on a sheet of paper. The patient colors in the area(s) where he or she hurts.

Other tests are often recommended, such as the tilt-table test for evaluating the autonomic nervous system. That's the part of the peripheral nervous system responsible for regulating various organs and functions, including blood pressure.

Fibromyalgia and Bipolar Disorder (BPD)

The psychological condition bipolar disorder, once known as manic depression, affects anywhere from 1.5 percent to 4 percent of adults. People with this mood disorder alternate between dark depression and episodes of hyper, impulsive behavior, or mania. Because depression is the dominant symptom, bipolar disorder is all too frequently misdiagnosed as simple depression, and the two conditions call for different treatments. According to one survey of BPD patients, it took nearly nine years, on average, for their condition to be diagnosed accurately.

While many professional reviews claim that bipolar disorder is rare in fibromyalgia patients, about 25 percent of my patients show evidence of this disorder based on their responses to the Mood Disorders Questionnaire (MDQ). So I ask all my patients to fill out the MDQ before a course of treatment is determined. It is important to know not only whether the person I am treating is depressed but also whether that person suffers from bipolar disorder.

A second reason why it's vital for me to know if a fibromyalgia patient also suffers from bipolar disorder as opposed to depression is that one treatment option for depression in patients with fibromyalgia includes the use of selective serotonin reuptake inhibitors (discussed in chapter 5). SSRIs have the potential to trigger an attack of mania in someone with undiagnosed bipolar disorder; therefore, these patients may need other classes of drugs to treat their depression.

The autonomic nervous system is subdivided into the sympathetic and parasympathetic nervous systems. Put simply, the sympathetic nerves rev us up to contend with life's stresses, by increasing our heart rate, boosting our blood pressure, and shunting blood to the skeletal muscles, heart, and brain, among other effects. In contrast, the parasympathetic nerves act to reverse the so-called fight-or-flight response and calm us down.

Autonomic dysfunction is common in fibromyalgia. It is characterized by too much sympathetic activity and too little parasympathetic activity. About one in five to three in five people with the disorder will experience low blood pressure in the veins charged with returning blood to the heart and lungs, where it picks up fresh oxygen. Low venous pressure may cause a person to feel light-headed or faint when sitting up suddenly. The tilt-table test calls for the patient to lie on his or her back on a mechanized table, which is then raised to a roughly 70-degree angle for 30 minutes or more, or until the patient experiences an abnormal drop in blood pressure. Men and women found to have this condition are typically treated with simple measures such as increasing the amount of salt in their diet or prescribing blood pressure medication.

Over the years, I've come to rely on these measures and tests, but I remain interested and open minded about the use of any other instrument that can help me and other doctors to improve our understanding of and treatment of fibromyalgia.

We've left Elaine sitting in my office without a final wrap-up. Let's go back.

Figure 2.3—FIQ Scales

The FIQ Directions and Questions

Directions: For questions 1 through 3, please circle the number that best describes how you did overall for the past week. If you don't normally do something that is asked, cross the question out.

Question 1.

Were you able to:	Always	Most of the time	Occasionally	Never
1. Do shopping?	0	1	2	3
2. Do laundry with washer and dryer?	0	1	2	3
3. Prepare meals?	0	1	2	3
4. Wash dishes/cooking utensils by hand?	0	1	2	3
5. Vacuum a rug?	0	1	2	3
6. Make beds?	0	1	2	3
7. Walk several blocks?	0	1	2	3
8. Visit friends or relatives?	0	1	2	3
9. Do yard work?	0	1	2	3
10. Drive a car?	0	1	2	3
11. Climb stairs?	0	1	2	3

Question 2. *Of the 7 days in the past week, how many days did you feel good?*

0   1   2   3   4   5   6   7

Question 3. *How many days last week did you miss work, including housework, because of your symptoms?*

0   1   2   3   4   5   6   7

Directions: For the remaining items, mark the point on the line that best indicates how you felt overall for the past week.

Question 4. *When you worked, how much did pain or other symptoms interfere with your ability to do your work, including housework?*

0   1   2   3   4   5   6   7   8   9   10

No problem with work   **Great difficulty with work**

Question 5. *How bad has your pain been?*

0   1   2   3   4   5   6   7   8   9   10

No pain   **Very severe pain**

Question 6. *How tired have you been?*

0   1   2   3   4   5   6   7   8   9   10

No tiredness   **Very tired**

Question 7. *How have you felt when you get up in the morning?*

0   1   2   3   4   5   6   7   8   9   10

Awoke well rested   **Awoke very tired**

Question 8. *How bad has your stiffness been?*

0   1   2   3   4   5   6   7   8   9   10

No stiffness   **Very stiff**

Question 9. *How nervous or anxious have you felt?*

0   1   2   3   4   5   6   7   8   9   10

Not anxious   **Very anxious**

Question 10. *How depressed or blue have you felt?*

0   1   2   3   4   5   6   7   8   9   10

Not depressed   **Very depressed**

As you can see in figure 2.3, Elaine has all the symptoms associated with fibromyalgia, and these symptoms are severe. From the way she filled out the FIQ scales, pain and fatigue are her most prominent symptoms. Her FIQ-DI score is 21/33, indicating that these symptoms are making life difficult for her to manage. From her SIS, I could see that her RPS was 16 and her FS was 8.

She filled out the Beck Depression Index and her calculated score was 31 points. People without depression usually score around 5 points. A score of 10 or above suggests mild depression. Her score indicates pretty severe depression.

Her MDQ score was 3. (See figure 2.4.) People with bipolar disorder usually score 7 or above, so Elaine's score falls in the normal range and is not indicative of bipolar disorder.

She also completed the Epworth Sleepinesss Scale, which has a possible total score of 24. (See figure 2.5.) The ESS test helps me differentiate "fatigue" from "low energy." Elaine already mentioned that her energy was low and that she was losing sleep, so her low score of 3 was not a surprise.

Based on these results, her history, my physical exam, and her symptom of recent aversion to noise and odors, my preliminary diagnosis was depression and stress resulting in central sensitization syndrome manifesting as fibromyalgia.

Elaine's next question, of course, was "What can be done to help me?" We'll talk about her treatment after we spend a little time talking about diseases that mimic fibromyalgia in chapter 3. And we'll detour to the science lab in chapter 4 to check out the physiological and chemical links between the body's function and fibromyalgia.

Figure 2.4—MDQ Score

THE MOOD DISORDER QUESTIONNAIRE
(#1–3)*

Instructions: Please answer each question to the best of your ability.

	YES	NO
1. Has there ever been a period of time when you were not your usual self and...		
...you felt so good or so hyper that other people thought you were not your normal self or you were so hyper that you got into trouble?	O	O
...you were so irritable that you shouted at people or started fights or arguments?	O	O
...you felt much more self-confident than usual?	O	O
...you got much less sleep than usual and found you didn't really miss it?	O	O
...you were much more talkative or spoke much faster than usual?	O	O
...thoughts raced through your head or you couldn't slow your mind down?	O	O
...you were so easily distracted by things around you that you had trouble concentrating or staying on track?	O	O
...you had much more energy than usual?	O	O
...you were much more active or did many more things than usual?	O	O
...you were much more social or outgoing than usual, for example, you telephoned friends in the middle of the night?	O	O
...you were much more interested in sex than usual?	O	O
...you did things that were unusual for you or that other people might have thought were excessive, foolish, or risky?	O	O
...spending money got you or your family into trouble?	O	O
2. If you checked YES to more than one of the above, have several of these ever happened during the same period of time?	O	O
3. How much of a problem did any of these cause you—like being unable to work; having family, money or legal troubles; getting into arguments or fights? *Please circle one response only.*		

No Problem   Minor Problem   Moderate Problem   Serious Problem

How Is Sleep Related to Fibromyalgia? Most of us think of sleep as a passive process that occurs when we "turn off" for a period of time each day. In fact, sleep is anything but passive. Your eyes move. Your muscle tone changes. Your brain remains active. And the activities of all three change as you progress through the two phases of sleep: rapid eye moment sleep, or REM sleep; and non-REM sleep, which is divided into four stages, for a total of five.

How much REM sleep and non-REM sleep you get, and in what percentages, contribute to whether you feel rested and refreshed after sleeping.

Figure 2.5—*Epworth Sleepiness Scale*

Epworth Sleepiness Scale

The Epworth Sleepiness Scale is used to determine the level of daytime sleepiness. Use the following scale to choose the most appropriate number for each situation:

0 = would *never* doze or sleep
1 = *slight* chance of dozing or sleeping
2 = *moderate* chance of dozing or sleeping
3 = *high* chance of dozing or sleeping

Fill out the following checklist to find out your score.

Situation	Chance of Dozing or Sleeping
Sitting and reading	_____
Watching television	_____
Sitting inactive in a public place	_____
Being a passenger in a motor vehicle for an hour or more	_____
Lying down in the afternoon	_____
Sitting and talking to someone	_____
Sitting quietly after lunch (no alcohol)	_____
Stopped for a few minutes in traffic while driving	_____
Total score (add the scores) (This is your Epworth score)	_____

Stage I and stage II non-REM sleep are light stages of sleep, where the body is preparing to enter deeper sleep.

Stages III and IV non-REM sleep are known as slow-wave sleep or delta-wave sleep. This kind of deep, rhythmic sleep makes up about 20 percent of a night's rest. The four stages of non-REM sleep lasts about 90 to 120 minutes.

Interestingly a normal sleep cycle begins with stage I non-REM sleep followed by stages II, III and IV, and then *back* to stages III and then II before entering the REM phase. These five stages repeat about five times during a normal night's sleep.

REM phase is an active phase of sleep, the one in which dreaming occurs. Eye movement and brain activity are heightened during REM sleep, while muscles are almost immobile.

Why is this important to fibromyalgia?

Because fibromyalgia is almost always accompanied by sleep disturbance. You get the most slow-wave sleep early in the sleep cycle, whereas REM sleep lasts longest later in

Common Sleep Disorders

- **Sleep apnea:** a serious sleep disturbance. In addition to snoring, men and women with the disorder may go for 20 to 30 seconds without breathing.

- **Narcolepsy:** a sleep disorder in which sleep intrudes upon wakefulness, and wakefulness intrudes upon sleep. Narcoleptics complain of feeling sleepy during the day and may actually fall asleep.

- **Restless legs syndrome (RLS):** believed to stem from a brain-chemical imbalance. People with RLS involuntarily move their legs while they are resting, especially at night, making sleep hard to come by.

the sleep cycle. During each stage, different brain chemicals, called neurotransmitters, are produced; they influence pain, fatigue, and quality of sleep. Stress, the environment, psychological conditions such as anxiety or depression, certain medications, and illness can disrupt the quality of refreshed sleep. On the other hand, we have medications that can improve the quality of sleep.

An important study in 1975 showed that electrical brain rhythms known as delta waves were absent or disrupted in fibromyalgia patients, and as a result, slow-wave sleep was deficient. A subsequent study demonstrated that when the slow-wave stage of sleep is interrupted, muscle tenderness increases and people complain of fatigue, loss of appetite, and a heavy sensation in their arms and legs—features much like those of fibromyalgia. Once they are able to enjoy normal slow-wave sleep, the symptoms subside. Still other studies have found that people deprived of non-REM sleep experience fibromyalgialike symptoms.

How Does Poor Sleep Leave Me More Than Just Tired?
Neurotransmitters factor in the connection between sleep and fibromyalgia. During non-REM sleep, for example, the neurotransmitter serotonin is produced, whereas production of the neurotransmitter norepinephrine is related to REM sleep.

When your sleep cycle is disrupted, the levels of neurotransmitters produced will also be disrupted. Research shows that sleep disruption influences how we perceive pain and is linked to certain conditions that often coexist with fibromyalgia.

For example, in studies of animals, lower levels of serotonin have been associated with increased sensitivity to pain. Other studies conclude that serotonin affects the pain-blocking properties of a natural morphinelike body chemical called endorphin. Consequently, when a drug that inhibited serotonin's action was used as a possible sleep aid, researchers found that some patients showed extreme sensitivity to pain. Scientists have also discovered that fibromyalgia patients have low levels of tryptophan, one of the building blocks of serotonin.

The connections are striking and leave little doubt that a lack of serotonin, produced during non-REM sleep, increases sensitivity to pain. In other words, when the body does not have the right chemical balance, the result in some people can be a state of hypersensitivity to pain.

One logical conclusion from the above information would be that people with fibromyalgia have low levels of endorphin. However, a small study of 11 women showed just the opposite: they had *increased* blood levels of endorphin compared with healthy people *and* rheumatoid arthritis patients.

Why is it important to compare fibromyalgia patients with rheumatoid arthritis patients? Because both groups experience pain. If the body produces endorphin in response to pain, then you could expect that endorphin levels would be high in the two sets of patients. Since endorphin levels are normal in rheumatoid arthritis patients, it's highly likely that some other reason accounts for the high levels of endorphin in men and women with fibromyalgia. Perhaps it reflects the body's attempt to compensate for low serotonin, although this possibility has not yet been researched.

Neurotransmitters also figure in the relationship between depression and sleep. Studies reveal that patients with certain types of depression don't get enough non-REM sleep and have low serotonin levels. Depression appears to deplete the brain of norepinephrine, which, in turn, prevents a person from achieving sufficient REM sleep.

Because psychiatric disorders such as depression often coexist with fibromyalgia, neurotransmitter balance may be a key element in the development of fibromyalgia.

HISTORICAL INTERLUDE

FIBROMYALGIA IN MUSIC, LITERATURE, AND SCIENCE

Is fibromyalgia a new concept? Maybe. But as you'll see, its roots reach back many years. References to symptoms of fibromyalgia appear in literature, music, science, and philosophy, with numerous famous figures from history believed to have possibly suffered from fibromyalgia long before it was known as such—among them Clara Schumann, the 19th-century German concert pianist; French novelist Gustave Flaubert; Charles Darwin, the father of evolution; English philosopher and mathematician Bertrand Russell; and writer Hans Christian Andersen.

For example, Hans Christian Andersen, born in 1805, is the author of many famous Danish fairy tales that remain popular even today because they describe common human experiences. Given his ability to speak to the common man, it is curious and telling that Andersen recognized the increased sensitivities of the noble class in "The Princess and the Pea" (1835). Andersen's father believed that he was of noble descent, and perhaps Andersen did as well. Perhaps, too, Andersen, who lived a solitary life and whose stories often dealt with loneliness and being different, experienced the same heightened sensitivity as the princess in the story.

Whether or not the author was writing autobiographically, "The Princess and the Pea" strikes a chord with many people suffering from FMS. There are numerous adaptations of Andersen's work, including an Italian version titled "The Most Sensitive Woman." Having taken liberal editorial license with the story, here is the "fibromyalia adaptation," with an epilogue:

Two hundred years ago, in a place far away, a prince, with the help of his mother the queen, was searching for a suitable bride. There was something lacking in every girl he met, however. Too tall. Too loud. Too fat.

One evening during a storm, a girl appeared at the palace door claiming to be a princess. In order to test her, the queen ordered a bed be prepared. A pea was placed beneath 20 mattresses, which were covered by 20 comforters. In the morning, the girl complained of sleeping badly and being bruised from lying on something hard all night.

The queen declared her a true princess, the prince married her, and they lived happily ever after.

Or did they?

For a few weeks, the couple lived in newlywed bliss. Then the princess, not accustomed to sharing her bed, began to be bothered by the prince's presence. After tossing and turning all night, she would wake up to the sound of the scullery maids banging pots and pans. Then the stable master's dogs began barking. It seemed that every morning the sounds got louder and more annoying to the princess.

"I can't get any rest," she moaned. The prince was at a loss. And, unfortunately, the prince was also at a loss when it came to the finer arts of marriage, so the princess's complaints were the only moaning coming from the bridal suite.

The princess was exhausted from her duties. She had to supervise servants and oversee dinners for a hundred huntsmen. She became forgetful and had no energy to do anything. It was all too much.

The queen was fond of boiled cabbage, but the princess couldn't stand the odor. She began having stomach pains and bloating. And if that wasn't enough, she had developed some sort of rheumatism. It didn't matter if she was sitting at the table with her ladies-in-waiting or horseback riding with the prince. She felt as if she had a toothache all over.

When she finally complained to the prince that she felt faint when she stood up, he called in the royal physicians to consult.

"You need rest, your highness," said the first royal physician. He prescribed a drink to make her sleepy (laudanum, a bit like morphine) at bedtime. It worked, and made her aches and pains feel better too. But it made her stomach pain much worse.

The next royal physician poked and purged her and did other shocking things requiring a nozzle, which didn't help her stomach pains one bit but severely damaged her pride.

The third royal physician concentrated on her aches and pains. He rubbed oil over her skin and then examined her. He vigorously massaged certain areas with such force that the poor princess began to cry. He prescribed an Egyptian plant called Colchicum autumnale *(colchicine) and willow branch extract (aspirin), which gave her diarrhea and made her stomach burn worse than ever. She stopped taking them.*

The fourth royal physician proposed to draw out a large portion of blood to stop her fainting and lightheadedness. The princess fainted dead away when she saw the enormous needle in the doctor's hand.

The last royal physician was an old man, seasoned by years of practice. He talked with the princess about her ailments and barely examined her at all. "I prescribe sunshine, fresh air, and exercise," said the doctor. "And hire a secretary to help run this castle. It's far too much for a lady of your sensibilities."

"How can I go on walks and ride horses with this pain?" asked the princess. She vowed never again to consult with doctors, although she did hire a secretary, deeming that sensible advice.

Over the years, she fell into a routine with the prince, which was pleasant, if not heavenly. Her energy and sleep improved, and she even began to ride and go for long walks in the fresh air. Truth be told, at times she felt almost cured.

Chapter 3

Mimics and Look-Alikes

I n this chapter we'll discuss two major topics: first, which conditions mimic fibromyalgia; and second, what happens when a person has both fibromyalgia and another disorder—such as an autoimmune disease or a debilitating fatigue syndrome—as is often the case. Understandably, a second condition complicates diagnosis and treatment.

It's important to note that fibromyalgia sufferers are no more likely than the general population to develop autoimmune diseases, in which the body's immune system misidentifies its own tissues as foreign and goes on the attack. It's the biological equivalent of friendly fire. However, men and women who've been diagnosed with autoimmune disorders such as systemic lupus erythematosus, rheumatoid arthritis, and Sjögren's syndrome face a higher incidence of fibromyalgia than the general population. Why? Because as we have discussed, stress is a major player in fibromyalgia, and people coping with autoimmune diseases are highly distressed, both physically and emotionally. When fibromyalgia is recognized and treated as a cofactor in lupus, rheumatoid arthritis, or Sjögren's syndrome, people feel better, and their quality of life improves.

That's one of the reasons why it's so important for your physician to look at *all* your symptoms and history. If fibromyalgia explains only some of your symptoms, something else may be going on. Unless it is diagnosed, you may continue to put up with stress, pain, and other adverse effects.

Conditions That Mimic Fibromyalgia

Without a doubt, the signs and symptoms of fibromyalgia can mimic those of autoimmune diseases. However, there is one major difference: many of the symptoms of autoimmune conditions are caused by inflammation, whereas the symptoms of fibromyalgia are not.

For example, a fair number of people with fibromyalgia complain not only of widespread pain but also that their joints hurt. Joint pain is a symptom of rheumatoid arthritis. Fatigue, which can manifest as weakness or lack of energy or even sleepiness, is symptomatic of fibromyalgia as well as rheumatoid arthritis and lupus. (See table 3.1 for more examples.)

How do doctors tell the difference? Sometimes, when symptoms and history warrant, an antinuclear antibody (ANA) blood test is ordered to definitively diagnose an autoimmune condition. The ANA test is useful only when

Table 3.1—Look-Alike Symptoms: Fibromyalgia or Autoimmune Disease?

Fibromyalgia	Autoimmune Disease
Pain and joint stiffness	Joint pain with swelling (rheumatoid arthritis, Sjögren's syndrome, lupus)
Sensitivity to heat or blushing easily	Rash from sun (lupus), skin redness (rheumatoid arthritis)
Light-headedness when changing position	Lupus
Dry mouth	Dry mouth and/or eyes (Sjögren's syndrome)
Muscle aches	Muscle aches (rheumatoid arthritis and lupus)
Fatigue	Fatigue (rheumatoid arthritis and lupus)
Depression	Depression (Sjögren's syndrome)

symptoms point to a particular autoimmune disorder; then the doctor can have a blood sample tested for the presence of antinuclear antibodies unique to specific diseases.

That's important because researchers have found that low levels of ANA exist in the general population, and many people—with fibromyalgia and without; with an autoimmune disease and without—test positive for ANA. So it is not an effective screening tool to "weed out" patients with an autoimmune condition from those with fibromyalgia. Nor is a positive result for a fibromyalgia patient necessarily an accurate predictor that autoimmune disease is present. The fact is, most blood tests that primary-care doctors might order for fibromyalgia patients are not useful and may only make it more difficult to diagnose correctly.

• • • Fast Fact • • •

The surface of a foreign microorganism carries proteins called antigens, which resemble proteins on one or more of the body's own cells. As explained earlier, the immune system erroneously launches a search-and-destroy mission against the body's cells, thinking that they're the perpetrators. This is referred to as molecular mimicry.

• • •

How Can Lupus Look Like Fibromyalgia?

Systemic lupus erythematosus, often shortened to lupus, is a chronic, inflammatory autoimmune disorder that affects mostly women between the ages of 10 and 50. It appears more often in African-Americans and Asians than in other races.

While we don't know the cause of lupus, some researchers think that it and other autoimmune diseases occur in response to an environmental trigger, such as infection. Symptoms of lupus differ from person to person, and, like fibromyalgia symptoms, they may come and go and range from mild to severe. Almost all lupus patients have joint pain, which can develop into arthritis (the kind that doesn't damage the bone around the joints), especially in the fingers, hands, wrists, and knees. Some of the general symptoms of lupus, which are similar to some fibromyalgia symptoms, include fever, fatigue, a flulike feeling, and muscle aches. Its signature, however, is a distinctive skin rash over the cheeks and nose that becomes worse following exposure to sunlight.

Like fibromyalgia, symptoms and history are important when making a diagnosis of lupus. Doctors look for the 11 signatures of the disease, and listen to the chest for heart or lung abnormalities. If a patient has at least 4 characteristics, lupus is considered as a possible diagnosis. Sometimes a chest X-ray looking for inflammation of the lungs or heart, or a urinalysis to check for protein, is ordered. The ANA test for antibodies specific to lupus may also be ordered.

At present, no cure exists for lupus; treatment is generally aimed at controlling symptoms. Researchers have found that people with both fibromyalgia and lupus are generally challenged by a poorer quality of life and greater difficulty performing daily activities than patients with either condition alone. In addition, people with both disorders usually must endure severe pain, fatigue, and headaches, and they feel sicker overall. They also feel much more frustration about their health.

What does this all mean? It means that people diagnosed with both lupus and fibromyalgia feel worse and have a poorer quality of life not because of lupus, but *because they have fibromyalgia in addition to lupus.* Fibromyalgia symptoms, as we've talked about, stem from stress—and in order to help people with both illnesses, the related stress needs to be treated appropriately.

How Can Sjögren's Syndrome Look Like Fibromyalgia?

In primary Sjögren's syndrome, the immune system attacks mainly the glands that make tears and saliva. Sjögren's syndrome can also arise against the backdrop of a rheumatic disorder such as rheumatoid arthritis, in which case it is called secondary Sjögren's syndrome.

About 1 percent of the population is affected by the primary form. Women over 40 are the group most likely to develop Sjögren's, which is characterized by dry eyes and dry mouth, although more severe symptoms such as blurred vision, difficulty swallowing or eating, fatigue—and, less frequently, joint pain—can occur. People with Sjögren's syndrome also have high rates of depression and sleep disturbance.

When diagnosing Sjögren's syndrome, we test patients' blood for autoantibodies particular to the condition. A test of the eyes, called a Schirmer's test, determines whether there is a reduction in tear production.

There is no known cure for Sjögren's syndrome, and treatment generally seeks to control and relieve symptoms.

People with Sjögren's syndrome are more likely to develop simultaneous fibromyalgia than people with other autoimmune conditions, probably due to depression and sleep disturbance, which the two conditions have in common. However, more people with fibromyalgia also have Sjögren's syndrome than one might expect, which may very well be because of the relationship between stress and the immune system.

How Can Rheumatoid Arthritis Look Like Fibromyalgia?

Like other autoimmune illnesses, rheumatoid arthritis affects more women than men, although it can occur at any age. It is believed that infection, genes, and hormones may play a part in rheumatoid arthritis, which touches about 2 percent of the population.

Rheumatoid arthritis usually starts gradually, with symptoms of fatigue and weakness, morning stiffness, and widespread joint and muscle aches—much like the hallmarks of fibromyalgia. Rheumatoid arthritis progresses to joint pain and swelling and can include anemia, eye redness, and pain, inflammation of the tissues surrounding the lungs (pleurisy), skin nodules, and numbness or tingling in the hands and feet. Joints on both sides of the body are affected equally, and symptoms can range from mild to quite severe.

While there is no known cure for rheumatoid arthritis, there is a wide range of treatment options, including physical therapy, medications, and, as a last resort, surgery.

Like Sjögren's syndrome, studies show that people with rheumatoid arthritis have a higher incidence of fibromyalgia than the general population. And people with both rheumatoid arthritis and fibromyalgia are more likely to be hospitalized, disabled, or experience complications such as high blood pressure, heart disease, or depression than those with rheumatoid arthritis alone.

Some symptoms of fibromyalgia, such as fragmented sleep, are common in rheumatoid arthritis patients. Morning stiffness, tender joints, and fatigue are more closely related to the lack of good sleep than to the inflammation of rheumatoid arthritis, which tells us that those symptoms are connected not to rheumatoid arthritis but to fibromyalgia. Some studies have concluded that people with rheumatoid arthritis and a past history of depression have more severe joint pain, fatigue, and disability.

Rheumatologists have learned from these studies that some of the signs and symptoms we blamed on rheumatoid arthritis were really attributable to fibromyalgia, and that knowledge has led us to change our approach to treatment. For example, we've found that prescribing antidepressants not only improves mood, it also improves sleep, which in turn helps moderate morning stiffness, fatigue, and joint swelling.

An important 2005 study by Dr. Dennis Ang, who trained at the Cleveland Clinic Orthopedic and Rheumatology Institute (ORI), followed nearly 1,300 men and women with rheumatoid arthritis for 18 years. Roughly 1 in 6 of them also suffered from depression. Dr. Ang and his colleagues found that the arthritis patients who were depressed were more than twice as likely to die at a younger age than their counterparts who did not suffer from depression. Their conclusion? Identifying depression and treating it in people with rheumatoid arthritis can extend life as well as improve symptoms. One logical explanation is that folks who feel depressed may neglect their physical and emotional health.

Other Syndromes and Fibromyalgia

The relationship of pain to stress and depression is not limited to autoimmune diseases.

Osteoarthritis is the wear-and-tear kind of arthritis that affects many people over the age of 60. One study of depressed people over 60 found that more than 50 percent had osteoarthritis, and that when their depression was treated, the level of joint pain decreased and the quality of life increased.

An even more interesting analysis helps us understand why some fibromyalgia symptoms occur even among the otherwise healthy general population. Researchers at University of Manchester tracked 829 men and women in a dozen diverse occupations for a year to see which factors were most responsible for pain in the neck, shoulders, or lower back. According to their report, published in Ann Rheum Dis, about 41 percent of those who reported *any* pain in *any* body location were more likely to be dissatisfied with their jobs and unhappy with their coworkers. Only 2 percent of the people in the study reported widespread pain—thus demonstrating that job stress increases the chance of experiencing muscle pain and suggesting that stress-related fibromyalgia pain can occur without having a full-blown fibromyalgia condition.

This is exactly what I have seen in my own practice over the past 34 years. People who complain of severe shoulder or hip pain from tendonitis or bursitis are far more likely to also have more life stress and poor sleep than people who come to me complaining of only mild to moderate pain. (Tendonitis denotes inflammation of the tendons, connective tissue that attaches muscle to bone; while bursitis is an inflammatory disorder involving fluid-filled sacs called bursae, which cushion and lubricate your joints so you can move without pain.) Furthermore, their pain from tendonitis or bursitis is more severe than in other patients; they often describe a burning or "electric shock" sensation with movement that is not present in other patients.

These descriptions make sense. The central sensitization of fibromyalgia is an issue of pain threshold; more nerves are firing than in someone without fibromyalgia. That accounts for why tendonitis and bursitis hurt more, burn more, and are more disabling than might be expected in someone who does not have fibromyalgia.

As we talked about in the section on autoimmune disease and fibromyalgia, it's critical to treat not only the tendonitis or bursitis but also the fibromyalgia symptoms in order to reduce and manage pain.

• • • *Fast Fact* • • •

In a Norwegian study, 57 fibromyalgia patients took part in treatment regimens that included aerobic exercise, cognitive behavioral stress management, or drug therapy consisting of low doses of an anti-depressant or a sleep medication before bed. The study measured the treatments against the severity of depression and found that the more severe the depressed mood, the less effective *any* treatment. This tells us that depression, a cofactor of distress in fibromyalgia, must be addressed in order to make treatment options work.

• • •

Mr. Smith

Mr. Smith had been referred to the rheumatology department at a university where I taught in the early 1990s, to evaluate his complaint of pain in every joint of his body. The pain was constant and worsened by movement or palpation. A sample of Mr. Smith's blood tested positive for three markers suggesting rheumatoid arthritis: (1) rheumatoid factor, an autoantibody frequently present in RA; (2), anti-CCP antibodies, found in up to 70 percent of patients with early stage RA; and (3) an elevated erythrocyte (red blood cell) sedimentation rate, or SED rate, which indicates inflammation in the body.

He'd been treated with medications that usually are effective in rheumatoid arthritis, but the drugs hadn't lessened his pain—and his blood tests still showed abnormalities. Now, typically, when rheumatoid arthritis is impervious to therapy, we'd expect to see some damage to the joints. But Mr. Smith's X-rays were normal.

I was asked to devise a more aggressive treatment plan for Mr. Smith. It was a puzzle. Truly resistant rheumatoid arthritis is rare. Between that and the absence of joint damage, it raised a red flag.

"Mr. Smith," I asked him, "do your joints ever swell?"

"No!" he said emphatically. "It's in the muscles. I keep telling them, it's in the muscles."

As you've already guessed, Mr. Smith had several other important symptoms: dry mouth and dry eyes, problems with sleeping, a lack of energy, and all the other indicators of fibromyalgia.

When I examined him, his joints and muscles were equally tender, there was no pain with passive joint movement, and the joints were indeed not swollen. In fact, he was tender to light touch virtually everywhere.

We looked a little closer at the blood chemistry and what specific antibodies were present. It all fit. Mr. Smith didn't need a more aggressive treatment plan; he needed a revised diagnosis.

He didn't have rheumatoid arthritis. He had Sjögren's syndrome and fibromyalgia. I see two or three cases similar to Mr. Smith's each month.

Two Tests You Shouldn't Have

Because autoimmune diseases can give rise to many confusing symptoms, some of them similar to those associated with fibromyalgia, doctors are often tempted to order a connective tissue panel. How does that help? Well, frankly, it doesn't.

Here are the facts. Roughly 0.2 percent of the population has lupus. The antinuclear antibody (ANA) blood test can be used to confirm a diagnosis of lupus. Unfortunately, up to 30 percent of the population can have a positive ANA test that does not indicate serious autoimmune disease. What this means is that only 1 person out of 50 to 150 people with a positive ANA actually has lupus. Not surprisingly, studies show that up to 26 percent of people with fibromyalgia *also* have false-positive (meaningless) ANA tests.

These studies caution that when a patient complains of fatigue, poor sleep, and chronic joint and muscle pain, these panels should never be ordered. Under these circumstances, the ANA test is being used to search for an autoimmune disease, not to confirm a diagnosis, and because of the high percentage of false-positive findings, it doesn't work well. It finds what isn't there and only confuses the doctor.

(continued)

On the other hand, if a patient complains of the following constellation of symptoms, an ANA test can help to confirm a diagnosis of lupus: joint swelling; frequent mouth ulcers; severe rash with sun exposure; low red blood cell and/or low white blood cell counts; and blood and protein in the urine, a possible sign of kidney disease.

Another test occasionally considered by some doctors when diagnosing fibromyalgia is a blood test for the Epstein-Barr virus (EBV). The U.S. Centers for Disease Control and Prevention (CDC) estimates that as many as 95 percent of adults between the ages of 35 and 40 have been infected with this common virus—a member of the herpes family—but they exhibited only mild, fleeting symptoms that may have gone unnoticed.

In some cases, Epstein-Barr progresses to infectious mononucleosis, which shares some symptoms with fibromyalgia, such as chronic fatigue. Some symptoms may last up to six months, which is called chronic Epstein-Barr, although laboratory tests seldom find an active Epstein-Barr infection in people with this form of the illness.

Remember what we discussed in chapter 2: most of the diagnostic "action" is in the history and physical exam. Laboratory testing is unnecessary, both to diagnose fibromyalgia and establish its severity, as well as to gauge a patient's response to treatment at subsequent visits.

Besides conditions that mimic the symptoms of fibromyalgia, a number of syndromes look and act very much like fibromyalgia. Let's take a look at some of these, including chronic fatigue syndrome, Lyme disease, Gulf War syndrome (post-traumatic stress disorder), multiple chemical sensitivity, and syndrome X. But first let's talk about somatization disorder.

When doctors are not knowledgeable enough about a particular medical condition and cannot find an organic cause for symptoms, they may settle on a diagnosis of somatization disorder—which means, bluntly, that the patient must be imagining the symptoms (according to psychiatrists, as a psychological defense mechanism). Such a diagnosis is also rooted in the physician's need to *give* a diagnosis and in the patient's need to *get* one. There's a lot of uncertainty in medicine, and doctors and patients need to focus more on how to treat the symptoms than on pinning a name on them. This would diminish the necessity of settling on an inappropriate diagnosis.

In fact, up to half of new patients seen by specialists exhibit symptoms that their doctors have not been able to explain using conventional lab tests. Often, specialists plug the symptoms into the framework of their particular area of medical expertise when making a diagnosis. For example, a urologist might diagnose and subsequently treat interstitial cystitis, a painful, chronic inflammatory disorder of the bladder, without considering that it often accompanies fibromyalgia. Similarly, a gastroenterologist might diagnose and treat the bloating and cramping of irritable bowel syndrome; an allergist, chemical sensitivity syndrome; and a rheumatologist, fibromyalgia or rheumatoid arthritis. Is each of these specialists studying only a small part of the elephant? It's entirely possible.

How Can Chronic Fatigue Syndrome Look Like Fibromyalgia?

Chronic fatigue syndrome first appeared on the medical radar in 1987, when an outbreak of suspected mononucleosis in Incline Village, Nevada, was reported in the *Journal of American Medical Association (JAMA)*.

The article reviewed the symptoms and results of laboratory tests and examinations of the 134 people affected. One by one, mononucleosis, Epstein-Barr virus, and other fatigue-related conditions were ruled out, and a new diagnosis, chronic fatigue syndrome, was born.

Outbreaks of fatigue have been reported since the 1930s. About 25 percent of the U.S. population experience fatigue lasting at least two weeks each year, and about 8 percent of patients in urban settings report fatigue that lasts more than six months without apparent cause.

In order to differentiate chronic fatigue syndrome from people who have simple intermittent fatigue, the criteria for chronic fatigue syndrome require (1) persistent fatigue for more than six months; (2) at least six symptoms such as chronic headaches, joint pain, muscle weakness, and widespread muscle pain; and (3) at least two physical findings such as sore throat, fever, and enlarged lymph nodes in the neck. Fibromyalgia patients often meet the criteria for chronic fatigue syndrome, and vice versa.

Some preliminary research suggests that chronic fatigue syndrome may be related to a serotonin gene different from the one associated with fibromyalgia. As with many other areas of medical research, new frontiers in fibromyalgia and related conditions are being discovered too fast for them to be included in the latest publications (like this one!).

How Can Lyme Disease Look Like Fibromyalgia?

Lyme disease is caused by a specific bacterium carried by the deer tick. This bacterium, *Borrelia burgdorferi*, can cause chronic infection in many human organ systems and give rise to a variety of symptoms. The bite of an infected deer tick produces a distinctive skin rash resembling a red bull's-eye in about two-thirds of Lyme disease sufferers.

Early symptoms include fatigue, muscle and/or joint pain, headache, fever, and neck stiffness—once again, much like fibromyalgia. Later on, patients may complain of swollen joints, among other effects. More severe symptoms can occur if Lyme disease goes untreated.

Doctors use a Western blot blood test to confirm Lyme disease. The Western blot test detects the presence of *antibodies* to *Borrelia burgdorferi*, not the bacterium itself. One of the stickier issues with Lyme disease is that you can test positive for months—and even years—after you have been successfully treated with antibiotics for 10 to 30 days, because the antibodies remain positive despite no evidence of continued infection.

The bacterium that causes Lyme disease can produce symptoms in many organs that mimic many conditions, which has led doctors to refer to it as "the great imitator." These symptoms include fatigue, muscle pain, headache, sleeplessness, and difficulty concentrating, and have the components of what we've described in this book as central sensitization. It's no wonder that Lyme disease and fibromyalgia can be confused.

One important distinction between Lyme disease and fibromyalgia is that Lyme disease is an infection; fibromyalgia is not. If a person has central nervous system symptoms such as fatigue or headache, and they stem from a bacterial infection such as the one that causes Lyme, signs of inflammation will be evident in the cerebrospinal fluid. This is the fluid that travels through the narrow channel in the three-layer protective membrane surrounding the brain and the spinal cord. In a procedure called a lumbar puncture, or spinal tap, the physician carefully places a long, thin needle between two vertebrae in the lower back and withdraws a specimen of cerebrospinal fluid. When analyzed in the laboratory, it will reveal a high concentration of infection-fighting white blood cells or specific proteins that indicate infection. A different type of fluid, synovial fluid, lubricates joints. When joints are swollen from Lyme disease, and we use a needle to aspirate a small amount of this fluid, it will test positive for inflammation. That is not the case with fibromyalgia.

Sometimes fatigue and other symptoms persist after the Lyme infection has run its course. Sometimes a person tests positive for Lyme even though he or she has never been treated for the infection. These two situations occur when people have had Lyme disease—or *think* they've had it—and may be identified inappropriately as post–Lyme disease. If tests reveal that there is no longer an active infection due to the Lyme disease bacterium, yet symptoms such as fatigue and headache persist, most physicians today agree that fibromyalgia is to blame and should be treated as such.

The group of symptoms called post–Lyme disease is no different from, and is treated the same as, fibromyalgia.

How Can Post-Traumatic Stress Disorder and Gulf War Syndrome Look Like Fibromyalgia?

Post-traumatic stress disorder. Post-traumatic stress disorder (PTSD) is defined as:

- Experiencing a severe stressful event;
- Reexperiencing the traumatic event;
- Numbed responsiveness to, or persistent avoidance of, stimuli associated with the trauma;
- Cognitive dysfunction (usually the inability to focus);
- Involuntary reactions to reminders of the traumatic event;
- Flashbacks, which may be akin to the disproved recovered-memory syndrome.

Post-traumatic stress disorder is associated with any past history of trauma, often along with anxiety disorder and/or depression. In one study, the likelihood of developing post-traumatic stress was most associated with the amount and quality of sleep at the time of trauma.

When patients with PTSD and fibromyalgia are stressed, they display similar changes in mild endocrine dysfunction as well as in regional brain blood flow. Not surprisingly, people with PTSD, like those with fibromyalgia, are likely to have a genetic "marker" for the serotonin transporter gene. In one study, of 77 fibromyalgia patients who were given the PTSD scale, 57 percent met the criteria for PTSD, indicating a high correlation between post-traumatic stress disorder and fibromyalgia.

Gulf War syndrome. Formal classification criteria for Gulf War syndrome have not been published. However, when statistical analysis was used to track symptoms of veterans who showed evidence of Gulf War syndrome compared to those veterans who did not, the symptoms identified as being consistent with Gulf War syndrome were fatigue, disordered sleep, headaches, and painful joints and muscles—also consistent with post-traumatic stress disorder.

Studies show that Gulf War syndrome sufferers also were diagnosed with knee pain, low back pain, and fibromyalgia (30 percent in each of two studies). According to a review of trauma-related symptoms of British soldiers during the Boer War and World War I, the prominent symptoms were diffuse body pain, palpitations, feeling faint, fatigue, and insomnia. In fact, these symptoms and signs have long been recognized as battle fatigue, shell shock, and combat exhaustion.

Of interest, the predominant signs and symptoms of Gulf War syndrome did not differ from the symptoms experienced by active service men and women whose illness was considered to have arisen from the Bosnian conflict of the mid-1990s or other past wars. The syndromes were very much the same, which argues against toxins or infections unique to any individual conflict and argues for similar causes.

It isn't hard to understand how these symptoms, typical of illness caused by stress, arise. Imagine being caught up in the accumulating misfortunes of war. Trapped in an unfamiliar land with no way out; fired upon randomly by hidden snipers or threatened by concealed roadside bombs. Facing death and, perhaps even worse, debilitating injury. It's no wonder that some soldiers suffer from lingering, unseen wounds such as Gulf War syndrome or PTSD.

This is not to say that all people with PTSD or Gulf War syndrome simply have central sensitization and fibromyalgia, but certainly a sizeable percentage of these people have every reason to feel distress, which predisposes them to develop concurrent illnesses.

How Can Multiple Chemical Sensitivity Syndrome Look Like Fibromyalgia?

No universally recognized classification criterion exists at this time for multiple chemical sensitivity syndrome. It is said to occur when an individual experiences symptoms in many organ systems after exposure to common, unrelated chemical substances in doses far below those established to cause harmful events in the general public.

What are the symptoms?

A 1994 study by two doctors from Washington State, Dedra Buchwald and Deborah Garrity, compared 30 patients with chronic fatigue syndrome, 30 with fibromyalgia, and another 30 with multiple chemical sensitivity. They concluded that symptoms of each condition are common in the others. That means that all three syndromes are very similar, though there are some differences. Let's compare fibromyalgia to multiple chemical sensitivity:

Table 3.2—Symptoms: Fibromyalgia versus Multiple Chemical
Sensitivity Syndrome

Symptom	Patients with Fibromyalgia	Patients with Multiple Chemical Sensitivity
Fatigue	83%	90%
Sore Throat	37%	50%
Diffuse Muscle Pain	97%	63%
Sleep Disturbance	77%	60%
Depression	33%	67%
Hypersensitivity to Pollutants, Smoke, Gas, Fumes, and Perfumes	67%	97%

Studies have found that patients with multiple chemical sensitivity may have an increased frequency of panic attacks and anxiety disorders as well as depression. So distress (stress) is an important factor in multiple chemical sensitivity. The similarities of symptoms and disease origins among people with multiple chemical sensitivity and those with fibromyalgia are striking, and the differences, trivial.

How Can Cardiac Syndrome X Look Like Fibromyalgia?

Chest pain (angina)—essentially the heart muscle's cry for help when it doesn't receive enough oxygen-rich blood from the coronary arteries—can be brought on by stress, extreme temperatures, heavy meals, smoking, alcohol, and exercise. Cardiac syndrome X describes a circumstance where a person complains of angina, but an imaging procedure called coronary angiography fails to find a blockage in the vessels to the heart. It is seen most frequently in women, particularly those who are premenopausal. Besides heart or chest pain, symptoms include numbness in the arms, shoulders, or wrists.

Two major studies show that cardiac syndrome X is caused by: (1) a disorder of the heart's arteries that are too tiny to be seen during standard tests such as cardiac catheterization; and (2) hypersensitivity to heart pain. Further theories hold that perhaps low levels of estrogen might contribute to syndrome X. Based on a 1995 report in the journal *Angiology*, about 30 percent of patients diagnosed with cardiac syndrome X also meet the identifying criteria for fibromyalgia.

Miscellaneous Relationships

Fibromyalgia has also been associated with attention deficit/hyperactivity syndrome (ADHD), myofascial pain dysfunction, and sick building syndrome, although the relationships are less well studied. What is known is that these diverse diagnoses share many of the same signs, symptoms, and other common associations: higher levels of anxiety and worry; more common among women than among men; and significant percentages of sufferers reporting that they'd experienced an adverse event before the symptoms emerged.

It's reasonable that fibromyalgia should be in cahoots with these conditions. After all, if the brain is too sensitive to light, sound, and so on, it becomes difficult to focus and concentrate, because you cannot filter out extraneous information—a central feature of ADHD. Patients with temporomandibular disorder (TMD) have tender points in the jaw muscles; I've observed it in all my patients with the disorder. Studies have found that people with TMD are very likely to have pain all over, and so myofascial pain dysfunction of the jaw's temporomandibular joint, too, may be a part of fibromyalgia.

Finally, the feelings of faintness, fatigue, and weakness encountered in sick building syndrome—attributed to indoor pollutants or germs in modern buildings with poor ventilation—are reminiscent of chronic fatigue syndrome and multiple chemical sensitivity. About 30 percent of patients with fibromyalgia or chronic fatigue syndrome have similar vascular abnormalities due to abnormal functioning of the autonomic nervous system.

Further research is clearly necessary, but including these conditions in the spectrum of stress-related illness appeals to me, and when I treat patients with conditions such as ADHD and TMD the same way I treat fibromyalgia, many improve.

Conclusion

Diagnosing fibromyalgia becomes more complicated when other conditions such as rheumatoid arthritis or Sjögren's syndrome are present. Symptoms overlap in many illnesses, and treating a primary condition such as rheumatoid arthritis may well improve *some* fibromyalgia symptoms. However, neither you nor your doctor should consider that to be good enough. If fatigue or sleep disorders or other symptoms continue after you've been treated for another condition, more investigation is needed. Similarly, if your joints swell and are painful after you've been diagnosed and treated for fibromyalgia, you know that something else is going on and you need to be reevaluated.

With so many similar conditions such as chronic fatigue syndrome, post-traumatic stress disorder, and Gulf War syndrome, it's sometimes difficult to pinpoint the exact cause of symptoms. That's where a thorough medical history can make a difference. If your doctor knows that, say, you served in Afghanistan, or are worried about losing your job, or are highly sensitive to light, it can help him or her find not only the cause but the best resolution for your particular symptoms.

Chapter 4

How Fibromyalgia Develops

In order to understand fibromyalgia, it's important to understand the science behind it, and to understand what causes it—and what doesn't. Remember that the more you know about fibromyalgia, the better your prognosis will be, so sit tight through this more technical chapter and read on.

The Sleep Connection

In 1985 my colleague Dr. Alan Mackenzie and I published a paper proposing a hypothesis that fibromyalgia (then still called fibrositis) had its origin in disrupted sleep, as had been theorized during the 1970s. We've talked about sleep and fibromyalgia, but let's dig a little deeper.

To recap, there are two stages of sleep: rapid eye movement (REM) sleep, which makes up one-quarter of a typical night's shut-eye, recurring roughly every 90 minutes, and non-REM sleep. The latter includes slow-wave sleep, a deep, rhythmic kind of sleep in which delta waves are produced.

Different brain chemicals, or neurotransmitters, are produced during the REM and non-REM stages. The neurotransmitter serotonin is related to non-REM sleep, and the neurotransmitter norepinephrine is related to REM sleep.

Why is this important?

Because neurotransmitters influence pain, fatigue, and quality of sleep, anything that changes the concentration of these neurotransmitters—such as stress, the environment, anxiety or depression, and certain medications—can decrease the percentage of restful sleep we get. Some drugs can actually increase the length of slow-wave sleep, which results in more and more restful sleep.

While you're peacefully drifting through slow-wave sleep, your endocrine system is mighty active, producing growth hormone and its cousin prolactin at their highest levels.

Dr. Harvey Moldofsky and his colleagues at the University of Toronto Center for Sleep and Chronobiology studied sleep patterns in fibromyalgia patients to confirm prior studies suggesting that sleep disturbance was a key factor in the origin of the disorder. We've discussed delta waves; your brain also generates alpha waves, an electrical rhythm that brings about a state of wakeful relaxation.

Moldofsky found that in fibromyalgia patients, alpha waves may be interspersed with or entirely displace delta waves (called alpha intrusion) during the restful stages of slow-wave sleep. The result is that fibromyalgia patients don't get enough slow-wave sleep, and what they do get is often interrupted.

Moldofsky also studied the effect of noise on restful sleep by measuring brain waves with an electroencephalogram (EEG). He compared the EEG results from when sleep was undisturbed with the results from when delta-wave sleep was interrupted by noise. Dolorimetry, a method of measuring pain levels using a spring-loaded instrument, was performed twice a day and revealed increased muscle tenderness after the nights of interrupted sleep. Subjects complained of fatigue, heavy limbs, and loss of appetite. But when they were allowed to sleep without interruption, their

What Is an EEG?

An EEG, or electroencephalogram, is a test that measures the tiny electrical impulses (brain waves) that brain cells use to communicate with one another. Typically, about 20 disk-shaped metal electrodes are adhered to the scalp with sticky paste. The electrodes' wire leads are then connected to an amplifier and a recording machine, which converts the brain's electrical activity into wavy lines and records them on a moving roll of graph paper.

An EEG can be used to help diagnose certain illnesses, but it is also used to identify sleep disturbances. Alpha waves and delta waves have distinctive patterns that are easily identified on an EEG recording.

slow-wave sleep returned to normal and their fibromyalgia-like symptoms disappeared.

In a similar study, this one from Denmark, healthy women without pain were deprived of REM sleep and/or slow-wave sleep. Only the volunteers who didn't get enough slow-wave sleep experienced fibromyalgialike symptoms. The studies showed, then, that people with fibromyalgia have disordered and deficient slow-wave sleep, and when slow-wave sleep is disrupted, it can cause fibromyalgialike symptoms. Conversely, the unwelcome effects disappear when healthy, restful slow-wave sleep is experienced.

What is the connection between sleep disturbance and the body's biological functions? That's where the neurotransmitter serotonin comes in.

The Serotonin Connection

We've talked about how serotonin is produced during non-REM sleep and briefly touched on the fact that serotonin is linked to how people perceive and feel pain. Animal studies have discovered that low levels of serotonin in the body seem to increase pain sensitivity and influence the effectiveness of endorphin, the pain-control chemical that is produced naturally by the body. Other studies have taught us that the level of serotonin produced is acted upon by the amount of an amino acid called tryptophan in the bloodstream.

Guess what? Patients with fibromyalgia have low levels of tryptophan.

Our connection begins to look like this:

Disrupted sleep → Interrupted slow-wave sleep → Insufficient non-REM rest → Low level of tryptophan → Low level of serotonin → Fibromyalgialike symptoms → Hypersensitivity to pain

It all starts to interlace, doesn't it?

One connection that takes a bit of pondering is why people with fibromyalgia have high levels of the morphine-like chemical endorphin. With a high level of endorphin, you'd expect them to feel less pain, not more. A study of 11 women with fibromyalgia showed just the opposite, however. They had increased blood levels of endorphin compared with healthy people and compared with rheumatoid arthritis sufferers, yet they hurt more. It's important that the fibromyalgia patients were compared to those with rheumatoid arthritis, because both groups experience pain. The logical conclusion, then, would be that *both* groups would have increased endorphin levels. This certainly suggests that something other than pain is at work in fibromyalgia patients. Perhaps the body is compensating for low serotonin levels. To date, we don't have the answer and need more research in this area.

The Depression Connection

Neurotransmitter balance, especially serotonin levels, is disturbed when a person feels depressed. Since we know that affective disorders such as depression are associated with fibromyalgia, neurotransmitter balance may well be a key element in the development of fibromyalgia.

Let's pull the conclusions together:

1. Depression or other factors disrupt slow-wave sleep.
2. Decreased slow-wave sleep results in lower levels of the neurotransmitter serotonin.
3. Deficient serotonin interferes with normal functions of endorphin.
4. These chemical abnormalities result in increased sensitivity to pain in normally tender areas of the spine and especially of the neck.
5. These areas of chronic pain produce the "pain all over" described by so many fibromyalgia patients. (A note of caution: the conclusion that chronic pain produces pain all over is only partially true. We'll get to the reason for that shortly.)

Over the years, many studies have found links between depression, psychological distress, and fibromyalgia. There is no question that many people with fibromyalgia have greater psychological distress than the general population, but it's important to note that about 25 percent of fibromyalgia sufferers have entirely normal psychological test results. However, the presence of depression and psychological distress, like other factors that play a major role in the genesis of fibromyalgia, *must* be treated before fibromyalgia symptoms can be addressed.

*   *   *   *** Fast Fact ***   *   *

We don't treat fibromyalgia.
We treat the factors responsible for fibromyalgia.

*   *   *

For now, it's important to note that fibromyalgia can result from a variety of sources, but, regardless of the source, the symptoms are the same. And in all cases, it is critical that your physician identify the factors responsible for fibromyalgia and address them during treatment.

For example, fibromyalgia can arise from or accompany:

*   Peripheral sensory conditions such as neuropathy (an abnormal or degenerative nerve problem), arthritis, and degenerative disease of the spongy disks between the spinal vertebrae.
*   Psychological conditions such as obsessive-compulsive states, depression, and other neuroses.
*   Pharmacological side effects and complications such as caffeine abuse, anorexia-inducing stimulants, narcotic withdrawal, and asthma drug therapy.
*   Metabolic imbalances such as low thyroid function (hypothyroidism).
*   And at least one paper has linked fibromyalgia to sleep apnea, a primary sleep disorder.

Joy

Joy was 36 years old and had been plagued with unexplained pains and symptoms for as long as she could remember. She considered her name quite ironic.

As a child, doctors had told her, "You're just having growing pains." All well and good, except that two decades later, she still was having "growing pains." These days, as she went from doctor to doctor, she'd tell them, "I'm sick and tired of being sick and tired."

The results were always the same. The doctors would say that her test results were normal and then diagnose her as having fibromyalgia. "Just fibromyalgia," most of them said.

They'd hand over prescriptions for drugs, but Joy was leery of taking medications, and so she didn't fill them. Once she told the doctors that she didn't want to take anything "unnatural," they usually spent less and less time with her. Along the way, one of the doctors told her to exercise and suggested that she'd just have to live with the symptoms because he didn't have anything else to offer.

Then a friend told her about an Internet site about fibromyalgia. Joy logged on and got the number for a new fibromyalgia clinic that had just opened in her area. She received an appointment for the very next day. The minute she walked into the clinic, she knew that her life was going to change for the better.

The waiting room was a quiet oasis. The lighting was gentle and indirect. The walls were a soft, watery blue, the furniture overstuffed and upholstered in pale greens and blues. Soothing oriental music played gently, almost inaudibly, in the background. The room seemed to enfold Joy, and when she was offered a steaming cup of mint-scented herbal tea, one word floated across her mind: perfect.

Well, almost perfect. There was that matter of a steep office visit fee she was asked to pay up front. Before she was offered tea.

In the examining room, an attractive middle-aged lady named Lucy introduced herself as Joy's therapist. Her voice was smooth, and she listened without interruption to Joy's tale of woe. She then examined Joy and found painful tender points on Joy's body.

"I'm going to order some tests, Joy," she said. "I believe you're having problems with your endocrine systems. Your pituitary, adrenal, and thyroid glands may not be producing enough hormones. We're going to look at your immune system too."

Lucy drew blood, and when Joy returned a week later—paying another hefty fee before she was ushered into the examining room—Lucy showed her the lab results from a very reputable local hospital.

A few tests were slightly low or at the low end of normal, just as Lucy had predicted. She wrote out a list of pills and supplements for Joy. Dehydroepiandrosterone, (DHEA) a synthetic hormone, for her endocrine system. Guaifenesin, an expectorant, and something to support her immune system. And several others, "all of which you can get at the new special health store just next store," said Lucy.

Joy had some nagging misgivings, but mostly she felt hopeful. Lucy never once mentioned fibromyalgia. She didn't prescribe anything "unnatural."

For the next few weeks, Joy religiously took her pills and supplements, and she did feel a little better. Then, just as her prescriptions ran low, the effect of the pills seemed to wear off, and she slid back to being almost as miserable as before.

"Maybe there's something else I could take," she told her husband. "I'm going to call Lucy."

Lucy was with a patient. Joy left her number. Lucy didn't call back. Joy called again. Lucy wasn't available.

"The supplements she prescribed aren't working very well," Joy told the receptionist. "And I'm a little confused."

The receptionist called back later that afternoon. "Lucy called refills in to the health store for you."

"But I really wanted to talk to her and see if there's something else she can do. The supplements aren't working."

"Lucy has done all she can for you," said the receptionist. Lucy filled the prescriptions, to the tune of $110, but they didn't work. A few weeks later, when Joy tried again to call Lucy, the number had been disconnected.

There *are* some unethical people who prey on patients with chronic illnesses. They mix in just enough realism, just enough medicine, to be believable long enough that they can collect big money from desperate patients.

But most people in the medical field are not operating scams. Doctors can, and sometimes do, miss the cause of fibromyalgia, though, especially when it comes to the endocrine and immune systems. Why?

Let's go on to find the answer to that question.

The Endocrine Connection

In 1936 Dr. Hans Selye defined stress as the body's non-specific response to any demand. Stressors can bring about reactions by the endocrine system and the autonomic nervous system. How? Take a look at figure 4.1.

Figure 4.1—*(Chain) Reactions to Stress*

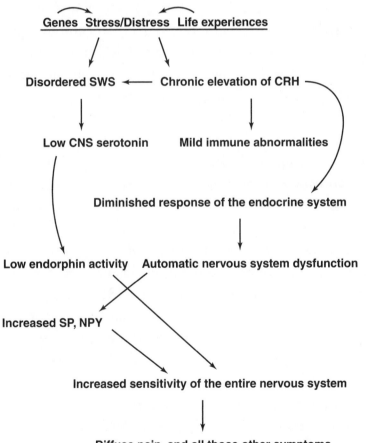

Genes Stress/Distress Life experiences

Disordered SWS ⟵ Chronic elevation of CRH

Low CNS serotonin   Mild immune abnormalities

Diminished response of the endocrine system

Low endorphin activity   Automatic nervous system dysfunction

Increased SP, NPY

Increased sensitivity of the entire nervous system

Diffuse pain, and all those other symptoms

Stressor → increased ACTH (an adrenal hormone) → increased cortisol (an adrenal secretion) → increase of epinephrine and norepinephrine (activate the flight-or-fight response in the nervous system)

You have two adrenal glands, one atop each kidney. Abnormalities of adrenal gland function can result in weakness, lethargy, low blood pressure, and an irritable stomach. The hypothalamus, a region of the brain, regulates functions such as food intake; it also produces and secretes corticotropin-releasing hormone (CRH). In fibromyalgia, chronic stress increases the amount of CRH in the circulation, which over time lowers blood levels of the hormone ACTH. The same thing happens with the nervous systems, often resulting in too much sympathetic-system fight-or-flight hormone or abnormalities in the parasympathetic system that produces tears, saliva, and allows for relaxation.

Eventually an overabundance of CRH renders the adrenal glands less responsive, with the net result a deficiency of norepinephrine. That's important because norepinephrine modulates the sensitivity of the spinal cord nerves. Not enough norepinephrine, and the nerves become oversensitized. In addition, abnormally high CRH decreases the relative amount of slow-wave sleep by a direct action on the brain. Put it all together, and the result is magnified pain.

At the very beginning of this book, I told you about substance P, which governs pain impulses sent from muscles and joints to the central nervous system by making the spinal cord more sensitive. The higher the concentration of substance P, the more pain a person feels. In two studies from the 1990s, the cerebrospinal fluid of fibromyalgia patients contained three times as much substance P than normal.

Substance P appears to be elevated when serotonin is low and CRH is high in the central nervous system. Serotonin is produced during the slow-wave sleep stage. Other studies have shown that people with fibromyalgia have lower concentrations of serotonin in their cerebrospinal fluid. See how it all fits together?

People with fibromyalgia lack a normal cortisol response. Cortisol, produced by the adrenal glands in response to inflammation, can inundate the blood during stress. It was logical, then, to study whether giving fibromyalgia patients cortisol (in the form of the hormonal agent hydrocortisone) might relieve symptoms. Dr. Robin McKenzie and colleagues at the National Institutes of Health did just that in a 1998 study. The results were disappointing. Some patients showed mild improvement, but the hydrocortisone treatment had no effect on pain. Along the same lines, thyroid and growth hormone replacement have been attempted, with largely disappointing results.

Pioneers in endocrinology recognized the importance of the adrenal glands in human disease. An absence of adrenal function, called Addison's disease, produces weakness, low blood pressure, and a poor response to stressors. Some early researchers postulated a new disease called hypoadrenia, or "a bit of Addison's disease." Such a condition, they theorized, resulted from diminished function of the adrenal glands and produced weakness, lethargy, low blood pressure, and gastric irritability, among other effects.

Early in the 20th century, a prominent physician named Charles Sajous postulated that hypoadrenia produced at least 96 symptoms—and so saying, many people with a host of nonspecific symptoms were treated with adrenal extracts, sometimes with initial success that was always short lived. Sajous's new definition of hypoadrenia included exhaustion, muscle pain, hypersensitivity to cold, cold extremities, low blood pressure, weak heart action and pulse, poor appetite, anemia, slow metabolism, constipation, mental fatigue, and decreased thyroid function. All of these signs and symptoms most likely indicated misdiagnosed fibromyalgia.

The Immune System Connection

The immune system, too, is linked to stress and fibromyalgia. For a 1991 study, researchers at Carnegie Mellon University gave approximately 400 healthy volunteers nasal drops containing a mild respiratory virus. Beforehand, the participants had filled out a questionnaire assessing their level of psychological stress. According to the report, published in the *New England Journal of Medicine,* the more stress that the subjects claimed to be under, the more likely they were to develop colds or respiratory infections.

Why might that be? Well, many other studies have demonstrated that stress may bring about depression as well as suppress the immune system. In fibromyalgia specifically, a variety of minor immune changes, such as a decrease in certain white blood cells, have been shown to help the body fight against viruses and provide other protective mechanisms such as cancer surveillance. The immune abnormalities might explain recent reports of a possible increase in the frequency of some cancers in patients with chronic, diffuse pain. The cause for this remains under study. Similar changes occur in chronic fatigue syndrome; hence the reason for the condition's earliest name: chronic fatigue immune dysfunction syndrome.

One possible mechanism is that cortisol response to stress is subdued in people with fibromyalgia. Two studies published in the American Medical Association journal *Archives of Internal Medicine* in 2006 concluded that sleep deprivation can be associated with proteins made by the immune system to cause inflammation. Linking inflammation to sleep disturbance adds another piece to the puzzle; sleep deprivation is yet another reason the immune system is activated.

The conclusion of all this is a simple but crucial point. While the endocrine and immune systems are clearly associated with fibromyalgia, endocrine and/or immune abnormalities are *complications* of fibromyalgia, not *causes* of it. The endocrine changes come about due to stress and related sleep disturbances. Therefore, treating endocrine abnormalities is not the answer; it's finding and eliminating the cause(s) of stress and poor sleep.

So Where Does the Pain of Fibromyalgia Originate?

In this chapter, we've talked a lot about how body systems link to fibromyalgia, but we've consistently stated that abnormalities in these body systems are not its cause. So what is? Let's start with the spinal cord.

One way to understand how the pain of fibromyalgia is felt "all over" is to appreciate the concept of referred pain, in which a person senses pain not only in the site where it originates, but in other body areas too. For example, heart attack pain is often felt in the left arm as well as in the chest and heart.

Another Reason Why You Hurt: The Spinal Cord

A landmark 2003 study confirmed that fibromyalgia patients are more sensitive to potentially painful stimuli than the general population. Dr. Jules Desmeules and his colleagues at Switzerland's Geneva University Hospital used an electrical shock of varying intensity to measure the nociceptive reflex in 80 people with fibromyalgia and 40 healthy volunteers. (The nociceptive reflex refers to, say, a stimulus traveling from a nerve in the leg, up the spinal cord and to the brain, which transmits a sensation of pain.) According to the study, it took one-third less electrical charge to the sural nerve in the leg for the fibromyalgia patients to feel pain in their upper thigh. Furthermore, the pain message triggered by the electrical shocks *never reached the brain*. This is important because it proves that the spinal cord generates fibromyalgia pain and, therefore, that nerve impulses amplified by the spinal cord is one of the mechanisms that make fibromyalgia patients more sensitive.

Referred pain hardly explains the other symptoms that accompany fibromyalgia, however. In the 1990s, research studies found that when pressure was applied to certain tender points, people with fibromyalgia felt pain, while those without fibromyalgia did not. Furthermore, two Australian researchers, Drs. Gerald Granges and Geoff Littlejohn, at the Monash Medical Centre, compared the pain thresholds of 60 fibromyalgia sufferers, 60 patients with chronic pain from conditions such as tendonitis and bursitis, and 60 pain-free volunteers. Their 1993 study concluded that the fibromyalgia patients sensed pain at a significantly lower pressure than the other two groups.

The Brain Connection

We've learned that the pain and central sensitization of fibromyalgia emanate from the spinal cord. The question remains, however, whether the brains of people with fibromyalgia respond differently to potentially painful stimulation.

Functional magnetic resonance imaging (fMRI) can visually show us that certain parts of the brain become more active when alerted to pain. Other studies with less sensitive instruments than the MRI have revealed abnormalities in blood flow to parts of the brain in fibromyalgia patients—even when they're resting. Much more research needs to be done in this field.

Another interesting study, this one from the National Institutes of Health in 2002, proves that although fibromyalgia is indeed "in the head," it is far from imagined. A small group of pain-free patients and fibromyalgia patients had pressure applied to the base of their thumbnails. According to the research team, when enough pressure was applied that both the people with fibromyalgia and their healthy counterparts felt pain, blood flow to the brain increased more in the men and women without fibromyalgia. However when less pressure was exerted—enough to produce pain only in the fibromyalgia group—cerebral circulation increased significantly in the fibromyalgia group but not the other group. Clearly, the brains of people with fibromyalgia process pain differently than normal.

The Myth of Hypervigilance

One psychological theory regarding pain perception in men and women with fibromyalgia is that they are "hypervigilant"—that is, they are more self-aware and therefore anticipate feeling pain . . . and then do.

As you've learned from this chapter, people with fibromyalgia are physiologically more sensitive to pain. There is a biological function responsible for how and why they feel the pain they do. If however, someone is psychologically self-aware (hypervigilant), he or she anticipates pain, and feels more pain each time that pain is applied in a gradually increasing fashion. In other words, if you apply minimal pain to a hypervigilant person, then a little more, and then still more, he or she begins to anticipate that when the pain comes again, it will hurt more than the last time, whether the stimulus is increased or not. The pain, in other words, is imagined.

For fibromyalgia patients, however, it doesn't matter whether the pain increases gradually or variably, in random fashion, it is perceived the same. There is no mental anticipation of the pain.

Central Sensitization

Increased sensitivity is not limited to pain perception in fibromyalgia patients. The autonomic nervous system, which regulates blood flow, the small and large bowels, the bladder, and the heart, among other organs, is also out of sync, or dysregulated.

For example, people with fibromyalgia have higher resting heart rates. When they stand up suddenly after sitting for a while, they may experience an abnormal drop in blood pressure, making them feel light-headed. They may also feel weak during or after a hot bath or shower. This shows that the sympathetic nervous system is overstimulated.

Sensory sensations, too, are often increased. Most of my fibromyalgia patients tell me that they are more sensitive to light, odor, and sound than other people. Investigators in Germany have shown that fibromyalgia patients find sound to be uncomfortably loud at lower levels than groups of nonfibromyalgia sufferers do.

One way to look at fibromyalgia is to consider it a condition in which more nerves fire than are supposed to when a stimulus is received. For example, when a sound is heard, more auditory nerves react, and so the sound *is* louder.

Where does this sensitivity come from? Is it genetic? Are people born with a tendency to central sensitization?

Fibromyalgia does occur repeatedly within families. For a 2004 study, a team led by Dr. Lesley Arnold of the Women's Heath Research Program at the University of Cincinnati College of Medicine collected data about tender points, pain intensity, and mood disorders in 533 relatives of 78 fibromyalgia patients and 272 relatives of 40 men and women with rheumatoid arthritis. They found that the likelihood of fibromyalgia patients' relatives having fibromyalgia themselves was 8.5 times higher than the incidence of fibromyalgia in relatives of those with RA. Mood disorders and pain scores were also significantly higher in the relatives of people with fibromyalgia.

This study, and others, strongly suggests that genes may indeed be calling the shots—but which genes?

The Human Serotonin Transporter Gene

The nucleus within every human cell contains 23 pairs of X-shaped chromosomes. A chromosome is composed of two coiled strands of DNA. Genes are located on these strands. An allele, one of two or more alternative forms of a gene, occupies corresponding sites on the two arms of a chromosome and determines alternative characteristics in inheritance.

The human serotonin transporter gene, located on chromosome 17, comes in two forms: a long allele and a short allele. These genes decode an important protein in the metabolism of serotonin and are typed as SS (two short alleles), SL (one short, one long), or LL (two long).

People with the two short alleles don't produce serotonin as well as some other people. Research has shown that they are likely to slip into depression, anxiety, or other mood disorders. As you know, these conditions often accompany fibromyalgia. Genetic studies found that the SS genotype was present in 31 percent of fibromyalgia patients as compared to just 16 percent of subjects without the disorder, thus suggesting that serotonin metabolism is an important factor in fibromyalgia. The serotonin transporter gene might even be a potential gene for fibromyalgia. Does it say anything else?

Ahmad Hariri is the director of the Pittsburgh Mind-Body Center, which is funded by the National Institutes of Health and affiliated with both the University of Pittsburgh and Carnegie Mellon University. He and his colleagues investigated whether the LL, SL, or SS genotype might modify the fear response. While participants looked at images of facial expressions that were happy, angry, or neutral, the researchers used functional magnetic resonance imaging to observe blood flow in their brains. For those with the LS or SS genotype, circulation increased in the part of the right brain that tells us whether to be afraid in response to an angry face. One interpretation of this study is that people may inherit their view of the world as a result of these serotonin genotypes. Those whose cells contain short alleles (SS or SL) see the world as a more menacing place than those with the LL genotype.

Conclusion

The contemporary theory of what causes fibromyalgia is a complex one that involves sleep disorder and diminished serotonin production, which in turn disrupts normal functioning of the endocrine system, immune system, and sympathetic nervous system. There is little evidence that muscle abnormalities play a part in fibromyalgia, nor does injury. However, genes and the level of perceived stress do play major roles. Our knowledge of fibromyalgia is still far from complete. The precise roles of the above factors and the relative importance of each call out for further research.

Figure 4.2—The Relationship of Factors That Give Rise to Fibromyalgia

Proposed Pathogenesis of FMS

"Distress"

past | experiences
genetic | predisposition
psychological ▼ factors

Sleep Disturbance

decreased | serotonin
"endorphin" ▼ insufficiency

Lowered Pain Thresholds

repetitive ↓ C-fiber firing

increased N-methyl-d-aspartic acid
↓
"allodynia"

Chapter 5

Conventional and Alternative Treatments

Therapy for fibromyalgia is carried out on two fronts: (1) treating the underlying causes of the disease—depression, anxiety, and feelings of helplessness—and (2) managing specific symptoms and complications, such as pain and sleep disturbances, and irritable bowel syndrome and interstitial cystitis, respectively.

One of the things that my patients want to know is, "What will my life be like with fibromyalgia?" It's not a simple question to answer, because people respond differently to treatments, and fibromyalgia patients often have coexisting conditions, which can make each case unique in terms of symptoms, treatment, and outcome. Most patients, though, will improve with the proper treatment.

Your individual prognosis depends on many factors. Learning more about fibromyalgia is a help. The simple act of reading this book has the potential to be a robust therapy for you!

In this chapter we will look at the common classes of drugs used to treat fibromyalgia and discuss why medication is only part of a treatment plan. We'll look at alternative therapies such as biofeedback and therapeutic massage, how best to use the Internet to gather information, and how to identify fraudulent treatments or clinics. We'll also talk about what you can expect from treatment, which as it turns out, is quite positive.

Let's start with the most complex intervention, the use of drugs in treating fibromyalgia.

Conventional Treatments

Medications

As patients, we've come to expect that there will be a drug available for whatever ails us and that we can just pop a pill to feel better. Television and magazine ads tout new medications and new treatments for everything from toenail fungus to restless legs. So it can be disappointing to patients diagnosed with fibromyalgia when they are told there is no magic elixir, no single pill, to fix fibromyalgia. Instead treatment consists of a multifaceted approach, a lifestyle strategy

Table 5.1—Generic and Brand Names of Drugs Used to Treat Fibromyalgia

Class of Drugs	Generic Name	Brand Name
Tricyclic Antidepressants	amitriptyline	Elavil
	doxepin	Sinequan
	nortriptyline	Pamelor
Selective Serotonin Reuptake Inhibitors (SSRIs)	citalopram	Celexa
	fluoxetine	Prozac
	paroxetine	Paxil
Serotonin-Norepinephrine Reuptake Inhibitors (SNRIs)	duloxetine	Cymbalta
	milnacipran	Savella
	venlafaxine	Effexor
Serotonin Modulators	trazodone	Desyrel
Serotonin Agonists	alosetron	Lotronex
Mood Stabilizers	quetiapine	Seroquel
Anticonvulsants	gabapentin	Neurontin
	pregabalin	Lyrica
Muscle Relaxants	cyclobenzaprine	Flexeril
Dopamine Agonists	pramipexole	Mirapex
	ropinirole	Requip
Anti-Parkinsonian Medications	carbidopa-levodopa	Sinemet
Anti-Anxiety Medications (Anxiolytics)	lorazepam	Ativan
Nonsteroidal Anti-Inflammatory Drugs (NSAIDs)	ibuprofen	Motrin
	naproxen	Naprosyn
Opioid Analgesics	meperidine	Demerol
	tramadol	Ultram
Sleeping Aids	sodium oxybate	Xyrem
	zolpidem	Ambien
	zopiclone	Zimovane
Anticoagulants	pentosan polysulfate sodium	Elmiron
Antispasmodics	hyoscine	Scopolamine
Central Nervous System Stimulants	methylphenidate	Ritalin
Miscellaneous	cimetropium	Cimetropium bromide
	dimethyl sulfoxide	DMSO
	perphenazine-amitriptyline	Triavil

built around reducing stress, increasing good sleep, getting aerobic exercise, and, yes, some prescription drug options to help with pain, sleep, and mood disorder.

Let's first look at physician-recommended drug treatments, which are drugs that have been tested in a clinical trial against a placebo and found to be effective. In the setting of fibromyalgia, many of these drugs are also used to treat depression because depression is often a cause of poor sleep and distress, and because some of the same central nervous system processes occur. These medicines, which increase serotonin and also, in some cases, norepinephrine, can benefit both conditions.

One of the initial drugs tested to treat fibromyalgia was a family known as tricyclic antidepressants, which are given in small doses at bedtime to increase the quantity of deep, restful slow-wave sleep.

Selective serotonin reuptake inhibitors (SSRIs) help the central nervous system to use serotonin more efficiently. Serotonin-norepinephrine reuptake inhibitors (SNRIs)—your doctor may also refer to them as dual reuptake inhibitors—help the central nervous system use both of those neurotransmitters. The three classes of medicines are logical choices to use in treating fibromyalgia.

Sodium oxybate, a sleeping compound sold under the brand name Xyrem, is a special case; it is a naturally occurring compound produced by the brain that increases slow-wave sleep. Although debate remains as to which mechanism is more important in fibromyalgia, most agents that alleviate pain enhance central nervous system concentrations of serotonin and norepinephrine, which decrease central nervous system and peripheral-nerve hypersensitivity.

Here is a table of other medications:

Type of Medication	Generic Name	Brand Name(s)	What We Know About It
SSRI	citalopram	Celexa	Has been found ineffective as treatment.
SNRI	venlafaxine	Effexor	Has been evaluated only in a small, 15-patient trial. In that study, 11 patients experienced some general improvement.
Serotonin Modulators	trazodone	Desyrel	Has been shown to increase the quantity of slow-wave sleep.
Major Tranquilizers	perphenazine-amitriptyline	Triavil	Studies performed in the 1970s on this and other major tranquilizers suggested usefulness in increasing slow-wave sleep and easing pain.
Anticonvulsants	pregabalin	Lyrica	Decreases nerve firing in the central nervous system and was shown to provide global symptom and pain improvement.
	gabapentin	Neurontin	Was shown to improve pain better than placebo.
Dopamine Agonists	pramipexole	Mirapex	A medicine that increases the effects of the neurotransmitter dopamine in the central nervous system, which may increase the relative amount of slow-wave sleep. Has also been shown to decrease pain versus placebo.

Although all of these drugs are used to treat fibromyalgia, only three, pregabalin, duloxetine, and milnacipran, are approved by the U.S. Food and Drug Administration (FDA) for this use. Other drugs have been shown to relieve pain and other symptoms of fibromyalgia and are prescribed "off label." That means they have won FDA approval, but as treatments of other illnesses, not fibromyalgia. Conducting the multiple phases of clinical trials necessary to bring a medication to market typically consumes hundreds of millions of dollars and is extraordinarily time consuming (almost nine years, on average), and so pharmaceutical manufacturers simply cannot afford to study a drug for every possible use. Over time, physicians often discover that a medication proved effective for treating one condition also benefits people with other disorders. For instance, the tricyclic antidepressant doxepin, an approved therapy for anxiety and depression, has also been found to improve slow-wave sleep. Accordingly, many doctors employ it in the treatment of fibromyalgia. Similarly, quetiapine (Seroquel), a mood stabilizer, was shown to improve fatigue in one study and can be combined with the anticonvulsant pregabalin.

Many of these drugs have been shown to work better than a placebo for fibromyalgia in drug trials. However, you must bear in mind that a clinical study reports the *average* improvement for the entire group of participants. Some folks fare much better than others. This is why drugs that are effective for the majority may not be effective for all. The question, then, is not just *whether* a drug is better than a placebo, but *how much better*. For instance, if a drug reduces the likelihood of a heart attack by 50 percent over a period of time, it appears to be effective. But is it really?

Well, *maybe*. Let's say that the group being given the drug under investigation is made up of healthy 25-year-old women. In this age group, the likelihood is that 2 women in 1,000 will have a heart attack. That's a pretty small ratio. So, for the drug to reduce the incidence of heart attack by 50 percent, it means that only 1 woman in 1,000 will experience a heart attack.

It also means that about 1,000 perfectly healthy 25-year-old women will take the drug in order to prevent 1 woman from suffering a heart attack. That is the *number needed to treat* for this drug. But some of those healthy women—say about 5 percent—will experience serious side effects from the drug; that is the *number needed to harm*.

Pretty apparent, isn't it, that a drug that saves 1 woman from heart attack but subjects 5 others to potentially harmful side effects isn't very good.

Are the Newer Drugs Better Than the Older Ones? The newest drugs used in the treatment of fibromyalgia are the SNRIs duloxetine and milnacipran, and the antiseizure medication pregabalin. Older SSRIs and tricyclics such as fluoxetine and amitriptyline, respectively, have been used for the past 20 years. Are the newer agents better than the old standbys? Let's compare:

Duloxetine (new-school)	Improved pain by 50%	752
	Improved depression "substantially"	60
Pregabalin (new-school)	Improved pain by 50%	602
Amitriptyline (old-school)	Improved pain by 50%	625
Combined amitriptyline and fluoxetine (old-school)	Improved ability to perform daily activities by 25%	178

The daily combination of amitriptyline (25 milligrams) and fluoxetine (20 milligrams) was superior for pain than either drug alone. The same was found for the combination of the muscle relaxant cyclobenzaprine (10 milligrams) and fluoxetine (20 milligrams) daily.

Other combinations have not been formally tested, but many of my patients seem to respond to a variety of combinations mixing any tricyclic with any of the SSRIs and SNRIs. Furthermore, these combinations are well tolerated. Side effects for most of these drugs are usually minor and include fatigue, dizziness, dry mouth, and constipation. Some should not be given to people with the eye disease glaucoma, severe heart problems, or prostate problems. A full discussion of side effects is beyond the scope of this book. Always ask your doctor about them when a prescription is given.

When someone has fibromyalgia and depression, we treat the depression first and then the causes of the symptoms of fibromyalgia. It's not because we can't treat fibromyalgia; it's because we don't always have the perfect treatment for depression—and until that's treated, the symptoms of fibromyalgia will continue.

How Do Drugs Used to Treat Fibromyalgia Compare to Placebos? Another way to understand effectiveness of treatment is to simply compare how well a drug reduces pain compared to a placebo. See table 5.2 for some results.

These analyses tell us what we know about lots of things in life: the newest is not always the best, although the newer drugs allow us to better tailor individual treatment plans. As an example of "old is better," the biggest improvement in

Table 5.2—Pain Improvement with Active Drug versus Placebo

	Percentage of Pain Improvement	
Agent/Dose	Active Drug	Placebo
Amitriptyline (50 milligrams)	20%	16%
Duloxetine (120 milligrams)	20%	13%
Pregabalin (450 milligrams)	15%	5%
Sodium oxybate (6 grams)	41%	16%
Amitriptyline (25 milligrams) + Fluoxetine (20 milligrams)	68%	−11%

pain was seen when amitriptyline and fluoxetine—a long-used combination—were prescribed.

The rationale for choosing these drugs as potential treatments for fibromyalgia was valid given our past and present understanding of its causes. The fact that they don't completely improve symptoms testifies to our incomplete knowledge of what makes fibromyalgia do what it does. Clearly, we need more effective drugs for depression. The effects of combining drugs for the treatment of fibromyalgia is also an area that is rich with possibilities for future studies.

Red Flag

Inflammation is not a component of fibromyalgia. Therefore, anti-inflammatory drugs such as ibuprofen, a popular NSAID, and the powerful corticosteroid prednisone (a dual anti-inflammatory and immune system suppressant) have little benefit and can even make fibromyalgia worse.

Nondrug Treatments

Exercise. The 12th-century physician and philosopher Maimonides wrote: "If one leads a sedentary life and does not take exercise, neglects the calls of nature, or is constipated—even if he eats wholesome food and takes care of himself in accordance with the medical rules—he will throughout his life be subject to aches and pains, and his strength will fail him."

Maimonides observed well. Exercise that is strenuous enough to improve physical fitness diminishes the pain of fibromyalgia. However, he did tout the benefit of "free perspiration," meaning that he was an advocate of aerobic exercise, which today is regarded as helpful for those with fibromyalgia. Study after study has shown that aerobics reduces the number of tender points and eases pain. I routinely recommend that my patients ride a stationary bike for at least 30 minutes 3 times a week.

Start slowly, with a short, moderate routine and gradually work up to vigorous exercise. The goal is to reach a heart rate at the low end of moderate intensity (that is 60 percent to 75 percent of your maximal heart rate) maintained for 20 to 30 minutes 3 times a week. Your maximum target heart rate can be calculated by subtracting your age from the number *220.*

We're not sure exactly how aerobic exercise helps. Some studies suggest that it improves sleep and increases the concentration of pain-relieving endorphin in the central nervous system.

Learn All You Can about Fibromyalgia. One of the most important things you can do to treat fibromyalgia is to reduce feelings of helplessness. If you know what causes fibromyalgia and what can be done to relieve the symptoms, you are more likely to develop effective strategies to ease your symptoms and respond to treatment. How can this be?

For example, if you have a headache but understand that it's a garden-variety tension headache caused by muscle contractions, then the headache pain is nothing more than a nuisance. However, say that you have the same headache, but you're worried that it might be a brain tumor. Then the headache rules your life and causes lots of stress.

The same thing happens with fibromyalgia. If you don't understand what causes its many—and very real—symptoms, then you might well imagine that you have any of a host of serious illnesses. You worry about it, your stress gets worse, and so do your symptoms.

How do you break the cycle and reduce your fear and helplessness? Reading this book is an excellent start, but don't stop there. Ask your physician for information about fibromyalgia and seek out reliable resources written by respected medical sources. You'll also find a number of excellent online sources in appendix I. One study demonstrated that ten weeks of weekly education and stress reduction helped fibromyalgia patients improve their ability to perform everyday tasks and activities. Cognitive behavioral therapy, which combines education with other stress-reducing therapies, is also effective.

Your pain can be reduced and your ability to function physically improved by an average of 30 percent when exercise, education, and stress reduction techniques are included in your treatment plan for fibromyalgia.

Alternative Treatments

After studying and treating fibromyalgia for many years, I have found most so-called natural therapies to be expensive and ineffective. Most doctors are practical people. If a treatment is safe and has positive effects on a disease, we'll use it. We are not automatically against alternative therapies—they just have to be proven to work.

For example, hydroxytryptophan, sold as a supplement, is a natural building block of serotonin, and so it made some sense to use it to treat fibromyalgia. Unfortunately, it got some very bad press when a Japanese company produced a contaminated batch containing bacterial toxins that caused serious damage to nerves and muscles. Many people who took the tainted batch suffered months of pain with movement (different from fibromyalgia), and a few died from untreatable nerve damage. Since then, the public has largely avoided hydroxytryptophan as a treatment for fibromyalgia.

Prior to this debacle, however, a study showed a variety of improvements in patients who took 100 milligrams of hydroxytryptophan 3 times daily compared to a placebo. Their pain improved by about half, and the average number of tender points fell from 10.5 to 6. Sleep patterns, fatigue, morning stiffness, and anxiety all improved significantly as well.

Hydroxytryptophan is an example of a natural, effective agent that *should* have been safe. Remember: "natural" usually just means unrefined. After all, what could be more natural than the poison arsenic, an element of the Earth's crust? Since the FDA has no jurisdiction and provides no oversight

for supplements (as hydroxytryptophan taught us), sometimes things can go terribly wrong. However, in 2007 the
FDA began to oversee alternative medicines to ensure that
the label properly identify a bottle's contents and that the
medication is free of contaminants. Perhaps this could again
allow the use of agents like hydroxytryptophan.

With that introduction, let's look at some of the most
popular alternative therapies for fibromyalgia.

Supplements and Hormonal Agents

S-adenosylmethionine (SAMe). The champion of alternative agents may be S-adenosylmethionine (SAMe), not
an herb or a hormone but a molecule produced by all living cells, including human cells. In some studies, SAMe
demonstrated antidepressant, pain-relieving, and anti-
inflammatory effects, the latter of which is unlikely to help
fibromyalgia. In one study, it reduced pain, but only by 5
percent—a barely noticeable improvement. So SAMe isn't
exactly a cure for fibromyalgia.

Super Malic. Super Malic is the brand name of this combination oral supplement containing malic acid and the
mineral magnesium. Biopsied muscle tissue taken from
some people with fibromyalgia revealed abnormally low
concentrations of magnesium. It was theorized, then, that
prescribing oral magnesium would replenish muscle stores
of magnesium and improve pain. However, when tested
against a placebo, Super Malic proved anything but, failing
to significantly reduce pain or the number of tender points.

Dehydroepiandrosterone (DHEA). A study of DHEA in 52 postmenopausal women with fibromyalgia showed no difference in any response versus a placebo, including the ability to carry out activities of daily living, fatigue, depression, pain, sexual function, anxiety, and mental concentration. This was true even in a subset of women who, at the start of the study, had abnormally low levels of DHEA.

Melatonin. The pineal gland, a tiny cone-shaped structure embedded deep within the brain, releases this hormone, especially when darkness falls. Melatonin, which is related to serotonin, regulates the circadian rhythms. However, more studies are needed to determine whether melatonin is effective at promoting sleep.

T3 Thyroid Supplementation. A study showed some improvement in pain, number of tender points, depression, and activities of daily living for patients receiving oral triiodothyronine (T3), a hormone produced by the thyroid gland. However, the number of patients was too low to draw firm conclusions, and no similar study has been conducted to date. The T3 supplement has been used as an antidepressant. The question is, could we be seeing an effect from improved depression, or, as I wrote in 1982, might it be due to improved deep sleep?

Growth Hormone (GH). People with fibromyalgia tend to get too little non-REM sleep, which is precisely when the central nervous system releases growth hormone. As a result, their GH activity is slightly reduced compared to that of the general population. Insulinlike growth factor (IGF-1), a related substance secreted by the liver, governs the physiological effects of growth hormone. When we test patients' blood level of IGF-1, up to half will be within the range of normal, but low. These individuals might benefit from intramuscular injections of growth hormone. According to one well-regarded nine-month study, women who received GH daily saw their number of tender points reduced by approximately 25 percent, and three in five experienced overall improvement.

Growth hormone, like thyroid hormone, falls under FDA regulation; the supplements DHEA, SAMe, melatonin, and Super Malic do not.

Miscellaneous Medications

Guaifenesin. This expectorant (an agent that thins mucus to facilitate effective coughing) has been touted on the Internet as a cure for fibromyalgia. It was claimed that guaifenesin corrected an inherited kidney problem thought to be the cause of fibromyalgia. The theory was that the kidneys didn't excrete phosphate correctly, and a buildup of phosphate in muscles led to abnormal contractions and pain. But a study found no improvement in pain or other symptoms when guaifenesin was taken twice daily, nor any change in phosphate excretion in the urine. Consequently, guaifenesin is not a recommended treatment for fibromyalgia, and the theory of how it may bring on FMS symptoms has been disproven. It may help you spit up phlegm, however!

Alternative Nondrug Treatments

Dietary Measures. These days, it seems like you can't listen to the morning news without hearing a segment about how diet affects health. Trans fats, antioxidants, organic food. Could there be a link between fibromyalgia and what people eat?

In one study, fibromyalgia patients on a strict vegan diet lost weight and had marginally improved pain. When a vegan diet was compared to giving patients a nighttime dose of the tricyclic antidepressant amitriptyline, pain improved in the diet group, but pain, fatigue, insomnia, and tender point count *all* improved with amitriptyline. Amitriptyline was clearly a superior treatment.

Natural chemical compounds (phytochemicals) called anthocyanins, derived from cranberries and blueberries, have been shown to improve sleep and general health. My advice is to eat fresh berries regularly. They taste good and in other studies have demonstrated some properties that benefit blood vessels and the heart.

Omega-3 fish oil has not been studied in fibromyalgia, but it has been shown in a carefully controlled study to ease pain in rheumatoid arthritis. Fish oil containing omega-3 fatty acids is one of the building blocks of fatty hormonelike substances called prostaglandins, some of which increase inflammation and some of which do not. Prostaglandins manufactured in the body from fish oil are *not* inflammatory. Remember chapter 3's discussion of how soft tissue pain from inflammatory conditions such as tendonitis and bursitis is often worse for men and women with fibromyalgia? Fish oil, which might confer other health benefits,

Because the world of alternative medicine is not rigidly regulated, to say the least, it's important to take precautions before seeking treatment. Appendix I contains the names, addresses, and contact information of the professional organizations for acupuncturists, hypnotherapists, and so on, to help you find a certified practitioner.

should reduce the pain of these local inflammatory conditions. Most of the healthiest fish oil comes from North Atlantic fish such as salmon and trout.

Acupuncture. Researchers don't fully understand how acupuncture works, but this ancient practice of inserting thin needles into specific body points to improve health and well-being is documented to reduce pain. It's logical, then, that it would be studied as a possible treatment to relieve the pain of fibromyalgia. The results to date, however, are inconclusive. An ambitious 2008 review of all studies examining acupuncture's efficacy as a treatment for lower back pain found it ineffective.

Biofeedback. Biofeedback uses electrodes to measure electrical discharges from the muscles coordinated with electrical impulses from the brain to allow patients to heed signals from their body in order to better cope with or improve their health. For example, to help relieve anxiety, the biofeedback machine might pick up an electrical signal from a tense muscle, which triggers a lightbulb to flash, signaling the person to relax. Over time, the response starts to become second nature. Chances are you've used a simple form of biofeedback yourself—such as when you feel your forehead to determine if you might have a fever. You're using your body's signal to feed back information, and then you take steps to improve the condition.

Biofeedback may help you relax, but does it work as a treatment for fibromyalgia? Three valid studies comparing it to placebo have been published. Two found no statistical evidence that biofeedback alone improved any symptoms. The third trial was entirely negative. However, when biofeedback was combined with physical activity, a modest overall improvement was demonstrated.

At this time, the evidence is not strong enough to recommend biofeedback alone. If it is used, it should be combined with an exercise program.

Meditation/Movement Therapy. Meditation is a form of focused, controlled attention or movement rooted in religious or spiritual traditions. It is often used as a kind of mind-body medicine, which proponents claim promotes health and wellness. But can it improve pain and the symptoms of fibromyalgia?

In one study, the participants practiced supervised meditation each week and daily home meditation for ten weeks. All exhibited some improvement, and 20 percent of them improved significantly. Another study compared three therapies: the Chinese movement therapy Qigong, medication, and education. All of the subjects improved, and none of treatments proved superior to the others.

Finally, in a trial of t'ai chi, 39 participants with fibromyalgia practiced the movement therapy for one hour twice a week. After six weeks, all saw their pain and fatigue reduced by approximately 25 percent. Probably more importantly, t'ai chi reduced anxiety and depression by approximately 35 percent.

These studies suggest that meditation and movement therapies might be appropriate for some patients with fibromyalgia, and I can't imagine serious side effects accruing from any of these practices.

Therapeutic Bathing. Therapeutic bathing, or balneotherapy, refers to soaking in warm water usually containing "medicinal" solutions such as sulfur, salt (such as from the waters of the Dead Sea), or other curative solutes. Therapeutic bathing has been a popular treatment for muscle and joint pain in Europe and the Near East for hundreds of years.

Three carefully controlled trials have shown mild benefit from balneotherapy for patients with fibromyalgia. In the best trial, the magnitude of improvement was small, with about a 10 percent improvement for treated patients and about 5 percent for untreated patients. Other studies have showed similar results.

Hypnotherapy. A 40-patient study compared stretching exercises to eight sessions of hypnotherapy. With hypnotherapy favored, the study showed improvement of overall pain, morning fatigue, sleep difficulties, and general well-being. The results may well depend on the talent of the hypnotherapist, though.

Therapeutic Massage. Fibromyalgia patients can sometimes find pain relief in the hands of a masseuse trained in techniques for this condition. Based on a few relatively small studies, it's not clear whether massage is effective in relieving fibromyalgia pain; however, I certainly wouldn't object to my patients trying intensive massage therapy for three months—and continuing it if they found it helpful.

Magnet Therapy. Testimonials about the power of magnets to relieve pain have been floating around for years, although the mechanism by which they allegedly work remains obscure. Do magnets measure up to claims? Based on studies, no, they don't. One carefully designed clinical trial, from the University of Virginia Health System, divided 119 men and women with fibromyalgia into five groups. For six months, two treatment group slept on magnetic pads. Two other groups slept on what they *thought* were magnetic pads, but were merely placebos; and a fifth group of patients received standard care. All five groups fared somewhat better than before in terms of pain and tender points, which tells us that magnets are no better than placebo, or no treatment at all. While magnets don't appear to harm those who use them, they aren't worth spending any money on, either.

Chiropractic Spinal Manipulation. Because fibromyalgia pain is often centered in the neck and upper back, there has been a lot of speculation about whether chiropractic manipulation of the spine can provide relief. Two studies examined the effects of chiropractic spinal manipulation. As with many studies trying to determine the effectiveness of certain treatments, they yielded conflicting results. Small but statistically significant pain reduction and improved functioning were demonstrated for a group receiving spinal manipulation versus a group receiving moist heat and standard care. Due to the small number of patients tested, further studies are needed before any definite recommendations can be made.

A Recap of Conventional and Alternative Medications and Nondrug Treatments

Shows Some Positive Evidence in Clinical Trials

Conventional Medications

- Amitriptyline or another tricyclic antidepressant in combination with the muscle relaxant cyclobenzaprine for sleep and pain
- The SSRI fluoxetine for sleep and fatigue
- The SNRI duloxetine for pain
- The SNRI milnacipran for fatigue and pain
- Pregabalin, an anticonvulsant, and the sleeping aid sodium oxybate for fatigue, sleep, and pain
- Tramadol (Ultram) for pain

Supplements and Hormonal Agents

- Hydroxytryptophan, a supplement, for sleep and pain
- Growth hormone, reserved for patients with low blood levels of insulinlike growth factor (IGF-1)

Nonpharmacologic Therapies

- Aerobic exercise for sleep, pain, and fatigue
- Education with or without stress management (cognitive behavioral therapy) for all symptoms

(continued)

Shows Very Little Positive Evidence

Supplements and Hormonal Agents

- SAMe—tested positive in one clinical trial, but the magnitude of pain improvement was very small
- Melatonin—fared well as a promoter of sleep in one study, but more research is needed
- Triiodothyronine (T3)—more studies needed to see if T3 can help ease pain and depression

Nonpharmacologic Therapies

- Biofeedback combined with exercise
- Meditation/movement to improve fatigue
- Hypnotherapy, provided that you find the right hypnotherapist
- Therapeutic bathing
- Therapeutic massage
- Chiropractic spinal manipulation

Shows No Evidence of Useful Benefit

Conventional Medications

- Guaifenesin
- Opioid pain relievers (analgesics)
- Prednisone or other corticosteroids
- NSAIDs alone
- Benzodiazepine drugs, or so-called minor tranquilizers (example: Valium) alone

Supplements and Hormonal Agents

- Super Malic
- DHEA

Nonpharmacologic Therapies

- Dietary measures
- Flexibility exercises (used as the "control" in aerobic exercise trials and conferred no benefits)
- Acupuncture
- Magnet therapy

Treatment of Syndromes within Fibromyalgia Syndrome

Sometimes people have what's called a dominant syndrome of symptoms (such as irritable bowel syndrome) as part of fibromyalgia. For those patients, treatment of the dominant syndrome should begin as soon as it is identified, even if treatment of other fibromyalgia symptoms is going well. Let's look at some of these associated syndromes and how their symptoms can be treated.

Help for Irritable Bowel Syndrome

About one in four patients with fibromyalgia have symptoms of irritable bowel syndrome (IBS).

Like the rest of the body, the bowel can be too sensitive when you have fibromyalgia, causing symptoms of bloating, cramping, abdominal pain, diarrhea, and constipation; the bowel feels full even when it isn't.

The most accepted set of symptoms used to diagnose IBS are 12 weeks of abdominal pain and discomfort, plus 2 or more of the following:

- Relief of pain with defecation
- Change in frequency of bowel movements
- Change in form or appearance of stool (narrow, ribbonlike bowel movements rather than bulky; or mixed with mucus)

Irritable bowel syndrome can be further divided into three subcategories based on whether the primary symptoms are constipation, diarrhea, or alternating constipation and diarrhea. Many treatment strategies for IBS have been attempted over the years. These include bulking agents, laxatives, antidiarrheal drugs that relax the bowel, antidepressants and new serotonin-enhancing agents. We'll start with the last first.

Just as serotonin is involved in the development of fibromyalgia, it plays a major role in IBS as well. The bowel contains serotonin receptors, which relax the undulating motion of the intestine when they are "turned on" by serotonin. Functionally, this system doesn't work well in people with IBS. Perhaps they have too little serotonin, just like in fibromyalgia?

A relatively new class of drugs called serotonin agonists, which includes tegaserod (brand name: Zelnorm) and alosetron (Lotronex), interact with these receptors and relax the bowel. Studies show that patients with any of the three symptom patterns, including diarrhea-prominent IBS, were more satisfied with their treatment than those taking a placebo. Unfortunately, tegaserod brings about severe constipation in two-thirds of those who take it. One out of eight patients experienced pain relief, but one out of seven suffered worsening constipation.

A similar trial has been conducted using alosetron. It should be noted that the drug was recalled shortly after being introduced in 2000, due to rare but severe side effects. Two years later, the FDA allowed it to be sold again, but with the following restrictions: "Lotronex is indicated only for women with severe diarrhea-predominant irritable bowel syndrome (IBS) who have not responded adequately to conventional therapy."

So while serotonin agonists offer some pain relief to all IBS patients, it's probably best reserved for those with diarrhea-predominant symptoms. Unfortunately, some patients treated with tegaserod have experienced heart problems, and the FDA has recalled the drug. We'll have to wait and see if it is reinstated in the future.

Another recent breakthrough for the treatment of IBS has been the use of tricyclic antidepressants. It seems that the drugs work through the central nervous system by decreasing the sensitivity of the brain's cortex (the part of the brain we use for thinking). How do we know this? Because doses of the drug used for IBS are well below the doses used for depression, and the benefits occur within days, rather than the weeks it takes for a tricyclic to improve depression.

Smooth-muscle relaxants such as cimetropium and hyoscine have also been used to treat IBS, but these drugs are not very effective, and laxatives and bulking agents (like Metamucil) have been found to be of little value.

A reasonable treatment plan for fibromyalgia patients with resistant IBS is to try nighttime tricyclic drugs. If your symptoms continue despite this treatment, it may be necessary for you to undergo a careful evaluation for other causes, such as celiac disease—bowel sensitivity to a component in food called gluten.

How Can I Get Help for Restless Legs Syndrome?

Restless legs syndrome (RLS) occurs in at least 5 percent of the general population and in at least 20 percent of patients with fibromyalgia. During RLS episodes, you have an urge to move your legs when you are at rest, especially in the evening.

Restless legs syndrome appears to be related to insufficient concentrations of a central nervous system chemical called dopamine. Similar to adrenaline, it acts on brain functions involving movement, emotions, and sensations of pleasure and pain. Low levels of dopamine heighten the activity in the cortex of the brain, which in turn produces the symptoms. Factors believed to be responsible for this problem include genetics (there is a high family occurrence of RLS), iron deficiency, depression, and sleep apnea. Unfortunately, antidepressant therapy, especially tricyclic drugs, can cause restless legs. This can certainly complicate treatment for a patient with both RLS and fibromyalgia. Relaxation techniques and aerobic exercise can be helpful additions. Drug therapy is usually necessary.

Before prescribing drugs, your doctor should order a blood test to check your blood levels of iron and a related protein called ferritin. If ferritin and iron are normal, and symptoms aren't constant, L-dopa, the precursor to dopamine, is an appropriate treatment. L-dopa (also called levodopa) is the mainstay for treating Parkinson's disease, and it also demonstrates effectiveness in managing restless legs syndrome, at least for some patients, on a short-term or intermittent basis. As in Parkinson's disease, patients are often prescribed Sinemet, a combination of levodopa and a substance called carbidopa, which prevents the medication from being absorbed prematurely in the bloodstream. You take it at bedtime.

Table 5.3—Medications for Restless Legs Syndrome

Agent	Dose per Day	Description
L-dopa + carbidopa (Sinemet)	50 milligrams to 100 milligrams	Probably best used intermittently because it may make the condition worse.
Ropinirole (Requip)	0.25 milligrams to 4 milligrams	A dopamine agonist; FDA approved for managing restless legs syndrome.
Pramipexole (Mirapex)	0.125 milligrams to 4 milligrams	Another dopamine agonist; not FDA approved for treating RLS.
Gabapentin (Neurontin)	600 milligrams to 1,800 milligrams	An anticonvulsant drug; works by decreasing the speed of neural transmission.
Narcotics	Variable	For short-term use, especially for treatment of augmentation.
Clonazepam (Klonopin)	0.25 milligrams to 2 milligrams	A dual anxiolytic and anticonvulsant.
Ferrous sulfate (Feosol; many other brand names)	325 milligrams three times daily	Ferritin stores iron. Ferrous should be prescribed only if your blood level of ferritin is below 50 micrograms per liter (mc/L); also, should be combined with vitamin C.

Unfortunately, up to 80 percent of patients who are prescribed L-dopa find that their leg symptoms worsen and start to occur earlier and earlier in the day. Should that happen, your physician would discontinue it in favor of one of the newer dopamine agonists, ropinirole (Requip) or pramipexole (Mirapex). Both are becoming popular first-line therapies. Common side effects include nausea and vomiting, sleepiness, fainting, and low blood pressure. About 30 percent of treated patients will experience at least one side effect. Any of the other drugs listed in table 5.3 may also be used in this situation, or, if initial symptoms are severe and occur daily, some patients may start with these drugs. It is sometimes necessary to rotate them.

Tricyclic drugs like doxepin can cause or worsen restless legs syndrome. Does adding one of these dopamine-enhancing drugs allow continued treatment with a tricyclic? Studies have not been done, and my own professional experience is too small to make any judgment.

How Can I Get Help for Interstitial Cystitis?

The concept of interstitial cystitis (IC) has changed over the years. When I first began practicing medicine in the mid-1970s, it was considered a chronic infection of the bladder wall and treated primarily with antibiotics. But times have changed. We now believe that the painful condition is caused by a loss of the bladder's mucous lining, which protects it from injury from potassium and other caustic substances. Under the old definition, interstitial cystitis was rare, affecting fewer than 1 percent of men and women, but using the new criteria, at least one in four people suffer from the disorder.

The characteristic symptoms of interstitial cystitis (IC) are:

- Pelvic pain and/or a chronic urgency to urinate
- Urinating eight or more times a day
- Frequent urinary tract infections
- Painful sexual intercourse
- In women, inflammation of the vagina (vaginitis)
- In men, chronic inflammation of the prostate gland (prostatitis)

Interstitial cystitis is diagnosed based on your symptoms and by your physician's using a catheter tube to instill a high–potassium chloride solution into the bladder. A patient without interstitial cystitis will not develop symptoms. But if the disease is present, it will quickly reveal itself.

Interstitial cystitis frequently arises as part of the syndrome of fibromyalgia. Dr. Daniel J. Clauw and his colleagues at Georgetown University Medical Center in Washington, D.C., sought to study the overlap of symptoms between fibromyalgia and interstitial cystitis. They enrolled 60 volunteers with FMS and 30 diagnosed with IC. When their signs and symptoms were compared, the two groups were more similar than not, generally manifesting all of the characteristics of fibromyalgia. (Anecdotally, most of my FMS patients complain of frequent urination and urgent bladder symptoms as part of their fibromyalgia symptom complex.)

The aim of treatment is to restore the bladder's protective inner lining. This is achieved by prescribing an oral anticoagulant medication called pentosan polysulfate sodium (Elmiron). Sometimes we additionally instill another anticoagulant, heparin (Warfarin), the local anesthetic lidocaine (Xylocaine), and sodium bicarbonate into the organ as part of drug therapy. You probably know the latter as an antacid. But for someone with interstitial cystitis, a doctor may use it to make the urine less acidic and thus less irritating to the bladder.

In addition, patients must restrict their consumption of foods rich in potassium such as citrus fruits and tomatoes. Other recommended interventions include the tricyclic antidepressant amitriptyline and antihistamines. Tricyclics actually *are* antihistamines, drugs that block histamine, a substance released by the immune system during allergic reactions. It's histamine that's to blame for hives, asthmatic wheezing, and other features of allergies.

I prefer to understand and treat interstitial cystitis as bladder wall hypersensitivity attributable to the central nervous system. Many of my patients with IC also have irritable bowel syndrome, and we understand that condition. In general, when I treat these patients for fibromyalgia, the bladder symptoms usually improve as other symptoms improve. For them, potassium damage of the bladder wall may not be the most significant mechanism.

If, however, all other symptoms respond to fibromyalgia treatment and severe bladder symptoms remain (a situation that I have yet to encounter), a trip to a urologist is indicated. That patient may have the "old" kind of interstitial cystitis, which calls for long-term antibiotics and instillation of a solvent called dimethyl sulfoxide (DMSO). Although DMSO has been tested as a possible therapy for assorted medical problems, to date the U.S. Food and Drug Administration has approved it only as a treatment for interstitial cystitis.

What about Relieving Sleep?

One of the most important symptoms to regulate with fibromyalgia is disturbed sleep. Until you are sleeping well and getting plenty of good slow-wave sleep, your symptoms probably won't get much better. You'll feel fatigued and stressed because you aren't well rested.

Most people report that they sleep better after starting an exercise routine. In some cases, medications are necessary to induce good rest. Benzodiazepine antianxiety drugs such as lorazepam (Ativan) and diazepam (Valium), and benzodiazepine sleeping pills like temazepam (Restoril), may induce sleep, but it's light sleep. The benzodiazepines actually diminish slow-wave sleep and, consequently, are not recommended for long-term treatment of fibromyalgia. Alternatively, the sleep agents eszopiclone (Lunesta) and zolpidem (Ambien) have been shown to improve sleep in fibromyalgia without reducing the time spent in slow-wave sleep.

Because the anticonvulsant medication pregabalin has been found to increase slow-wave sleep and does produce sleepiness, I sometimes prescribe it at a low dose (75 milligrams to 100 milligrams) before bedtime for patients who cannot tolerate tricyclic drugs or for whom the medications have not worked. Some patients appear to benefit.

Medication aside, there are many steps that you can take to help yourself get to sleep, such as the following recommendations from the National Institute of Arthritis and Musculoskeletal and Skin Diseases:

- Stick to regular sleep habits. Try to go to bed at the same time every night and get up at the same time every morning, including weekends and vacations.

- Avoid caffeine. If consumed too close to bedtime, the caffeine in coffee, soft drinks, chocolate, and some medications can prevent you from sleeping soundly— or sleeping at all. Alcohol may seem to make you feel sleepy, but having a drink around bedtime can disrupt your sleep.

- Exercising during the day can enhance nighttime sleep. But avoid physical activity within three hours of bedtime, which can be stimulating and keep you awake.

- Daytime naps may sound heavenly, but avoid them, because sleeping in the afternoon can interfere with nighttime sleep. If you feel you cannot get by without a nap, set an alarm for no more than one hour. When it goes off, don't linger; start moving.

- Watching the late news, reading, or working on your laptop in bed can stimulate you, making it hard to conk out. Reserve your bed for sleeping.

- Keep the bedroom dark, quiet, and cool.

- To avoid trips to the bathroom in the middle of the night, stay away from liquids and spicy foods after dinner.

- Wind down before bed by listening to relaxing music or taking a warm bath. (The bath will also soothe sore muscles.)

What about Relieving Fatigue?

I ask my patients to provide a synonym for fatigue, which can be an umbrella word for many kinds of tiredness. If they tell me that they have no energy or are "exhausted" and that they sleep poorly at night, I usually find that this means that they have depression or anxiety as the cause of fatigue and prescribe accordingly.

Fast Fact

Myofascial pain refers to regional pain in muscles, generally thought to be the result of remote injury or chronic strain. When the painful area is palpated, pain is not only felt at the site of palpation, but also in areas both distal and proximal to palpation. This palpated area is called a "trigger point." For instance, after a motor vehicle accident, a subject might complain of pain at the left side of the neck, and a trigger point is found in the left trapezius muscle. In contradistinction, the pain of fibromyalgia is diffuse, not regional, and palpation of tender points does not result in pain other than at the site of palpation. Effective treatment of trigger points include local injection of analgesic agents such as Xylocaine. This sort of treatment is not very effective for fibromyalgia, and this is why these conditions are separated.

If, on the other hand, they complain of sleeping too much and falling asleep during the day, I often find that they have a primary sleep disorder such as sleep apnea or restless legs syndrome, and treat these appropriately.

Stimulants are prescribed by some doctors to improve fatigue. I rarely use these drugs. Rather than treat the symptom, I prefer to treat its cause.

What about Relieving Pain?

Treating the pain of fibromyalgia is a slippery slope. The pain is the result of some underlying causes: stress, poor sleep, anxiety, or depression. Many people with fibromyalgia find that once those causes are managed, and exercise and education programs are put in place, the pain subsides. Still, pain relievers are necessary in some cases.

Powerful opioid analgesics such as meperidine (Demerol) or morphine (MS Contin is one of several brand names) do improve peripheral pain, but they are not very effective for the centrally mediated pain of fibromyalgia. They can also lead to addiction in a small number of patients, although most people with chronic pain will not become dependent. We know that when serotonin is low, concentrations of an amino acid called N-methyl-D-aspartate (NMDA) increase. The NMDA, you'll recall, boosts substance P production and directly stimulates the spinal cord, generating pain. Morphine acts on the nervous system to block pain, as does the local anesthetic Xylocaine. But neither of those drugs blocks NMDA. A general anesthetic called ketamine (Ketalar) *does* block NMDA production, and therefore works much better at stopping the pain associated with fibromyalgia.

• • • *Fast Fact* • • •

Your muscles are encased in a thin layer of
connective tissue called myofascia.

• • •

If I must choose a drug for pain, I use tramadol (Ultram) because this opioid analgesic acts in a unique way: besides enhancing the pain-relieving properties of serotonin and norepinephrine, it stimulates the brain's opioid receptors (docking stations, if you will, where opioid drugs attach to brain cells), which decreases pain. Yet another benefit: the potential of a patient becoming addicted to tramadol is lower than with other opioids.

Since we know that fibromyalgia is not an exclusive diagnosis, it's not surprising that many people with fibromyalgia also have so-called regional pain syndromes such as tendonitis, bursitis, or myofascial pain from past injury or overuse. In regional pain, the distress signals come from the body's periphery—the shoulder, for instance—and indicate possible tissue damage. These conditions can be successfully treated using over-the-counter nonsteroidal anti-inflammatory drugs (NSAIDs) such as ibuprofen (Motrin) or naproxen (Aleve).

• • • *Fast Fact* • • •

Not all people with fibromyalgia respond to even the most aggressive therapies. When they do, most effective treatments improve fibromyalgia by about 20 percent. The best approaches include effective drugs to treat sleep and mood, plus aerobic exercise.

• • •

The Wrong Sources

Excellent websites with great information about fibromyalgia exist on the Web, such as those run by the patient advocacy organization American Fibromyalgia Syndrome

Association and the online educational and support site the Fibromyalgia Network. But you have to beware when searching the Internet, because you can waste a lot of time and money. For example, this afternoon I surfed the Net using the Yahoo! browser to learn more about what it has to offer about the treatment of fibromyalgia. Here is what I found among the first ten entries:

- Emu oil for sale; promised that it would cure fibromyalgia "in 15 minutes."
- Oral hyaluronic acid (something a doctor might inject into an arthritic knee) for sale.
- Doctors' sites with ads for the expectorant guaifenesin.
- Multiple supplements such as shark cartilage and one site's own special brand of glucosamine.
- Various supports and braces, which could be appropriate for sports injuries.
- A variety of herbal remedies.
- Supplements to boost the immune system.

I investigated the academic backgrounds of three doctors who, according to their websites were international fibromyalgia experts. None had ever published an article in a scientific journal or was affiliated with a recognized medical facility. It seems that they had founded their own specialty clinics, which, of course, didn't require such professional credentials. Which brings us to a second warning:

"FMS Clinics"

How do you choose a doctor or clinic to provide medical care? One of the safest ways is to inquire through your local academy of medicine. That's a professional organization of physicians. Virtually all cities and states have one (our local, for example, is the Cleveland Academy of Medicine), and most provide referrals, often via a "physician finder" feature on their websites. I've included several other reliable resources in appendix I. Without recommendations from established resources, you are at the mercy of dubious practitioners on the Internet or listed among the newspaper and Yellow Pages ads for fibromyalgia clinics.

Rheumatologists are generally your best bet. What you want is a professional experienced in treating fibromyalgia. How do you find out? Call and ask! *Before* you make an appointment for a consultation. If the physician or someone on his staff says that he seen, say, 50 or fewer FMS patients in the last few years, try someone else.

Watch for these red flags concerning health-related claims made on the Internet. There are more, but these two rank right up there:

1. *If it looks and sounds too good to be true, it generally is.* If the clinic or doctor promises miracle results practically overnight, proceed with caution. If the clinic or doctor promises instant pain relief with a miracle drug or herb or treatment, proceed with caution.

2. *Even though you have insurance coverage, the doctor or clinic asks for money up front out of your pocket.* Why do you think they want payment up front? One probable reason is that these "therapists" know that insurance companies *won't* pay for the treatments they offer. The reason? Because insurance companies don't pay for therapies that are not approved or have proven to be ineffective.

In most cases, treatments offered by these doctors or clinics have been tested by reputable medical entities, and qualified evidence already exists to show that these treatments do not improve signs and symptoms of fibromyalgia. From the information we've discussed in this chapter, it's easy to guess what some of these treatments might be: perhaps guaifenesin, DHEA, or acupuncture, to name a few. These clinics or doctors direct their treatment at symptoms and don't treat the root causes of fibromyalgia. Their "treatments" may relieve symptoms or pain briefly, but the pain and symptoms are likely to return.

As we've learned, many people with fibromyalgia respond positively to treatment. Some do not. Symptoms can be controlled in most cases, but finding a universal "cure" that works for everyone, given the diverse illness factors at play, is highly unlikely. Patients who continue to endure severe symptoms even with the best treatments that organized medicine has to offer can become desperate for relief, and unethical entrepreneurs recognize a chance for profit. Be careful not to fall into their trap

Back to Elaine

Earlier in the book, I introduced you to a patient named Elaine, who had moderate-to-severe depression as well as anxiety and moderate sleep difficulty. I treated her depression with the selective serotonin reuptake inhibitor paroxetine (Paxil) because it is also effective for anxiety. To help Elaine get sound sleep and raise her pain threshold, I prescribed the tricyclic antidepressant doxepin, to be taken one hour before bed. Then I reviewed with her the key factors in the origin of fibromyalgia and how they can increase its severity. I encouraged her to return to exercise class with the goal of increased cardiovascular conditioning. This could be best accomplished using a treadmill or stationary bicycle.

All in all, it's not a complicated treatment plan, but it does address the underpinnings of fibromyalgia: stress, poor sleep, and mood disorder.

If I were to develop a treatment plan for you, it might not look quite the same as Elaine's. But it would be based on the same rationale: treat the root causes, not the symptoms. It would include a combination of drug therapy, exercise, and education, and I would encourage you to become an active, well-informed participant in your treatment plan.

Chapter 6

Controversial Theories about Fibromyalgia

There are many controversies surrounding fibromyalgia, ranging from whether it is a useful label for a real condition, to what causes it and what might cure it.

We'll talk about four of those controversies in this chapter:

- Is fibromyalgia is a useful label?
- Does abuse early in life cause fibromyalgia?
- Can neck surgery cure fibromyalgia?
- Is there a link between silicone breast implants and fibromyalgia?

Fibromyalgia as a Diagnostic Label

Fibromyalgia is a painful condition caused by central nervous system sensitization. There are physiological reasons why it develops, and there are similar conditions, and look-alikes, and mimics—all of which we've discussed.

So why do some doctors contend that fibromyalgia shouldn't be identified as a distinct medical condition? Perhaps because physicians are by nature conservative and have trouble integrating new information into deeply ingrained beliefs. Not only that, figuring out what triggers fibromyalgia takes a lot of listening to patients, and time is not exactly in huge supply in a doctor's typical day.

And what about the premise that a diagnosis of fibromyalgia leads to underrecognition or failure to treat the causes of the condition? Does a doctor sometimes overlook a mood disorder or stress when diagnosing fibromyalgia? While not frequent, it does happen. Doctors who may not thoroughly understand the physiological mechanisms of fibromyalgia can fail to spot one or more important causes. The harm to the patient isn't that fibromyalgia was identified, it's that the doctor might not understand the underlying factors in fibromyalgia, and so he or she doesn't look for or treat mood disorder, or stress, or poor sleep, and hence patients continue to be unwell. Having fibromyalgia identified as a syndrome with specific, identifiable symptoms and treatments helps *avoid* such issues. Furthermore, experience has shown me that, on the whole, patients do better once they know that their symptoms belong to a recognized medical condition with a treatment plan that can benefit them.

Fibromyalgia and Abuse

Is childhood abuse a cause of fibromyalgia? That question does not have a straightforward answer.

One theory holds that children exposed in infancy to pain (say, from a medical procedure) or physical abuse have impaired, or abnormal, sensitivity to pain. Two studies found that adult women with fibromyalgia experienced a slightly higher frequency of physical abuse compared to women with other painful conditions. Women with fibromyalgia also report a much higher frequency of sexual abuse, particularly rape.

Unfortunately, these studies are not as unbiased as we'd like. Many women in the studies used drugs or alcohol or had symptoms of distress. (Remember our discussion about how genes and fibromyalgia are linked to emotional distress?) There is a difference between associations (things that occur together) and causes here, and the interplay of extenuating factors is important.

Based on the data that I've seen, I don't believe that a history of physical or sexual abuse is a strong factor in causing fibromyalgia. On the other hand, a history of rape, especially when it has been physically and psychologically brutal, appears to be a significant factor in the medical literature and in my own practice. I also think that trauma occurring very early in life, such as medical interventions performed on infants in a hospital's neonatal unit, is an important factor.

Neck Surgery to Cure Fibromyalgia

On March 10, 2000, I was at a restaurant in San Diego with other rheumatologists for a meeting when the television news program *20/20* came on the air. In one segment, hosted by Dr. Timothy Johnson, neurosurgeons Michael Rosner and Dan Heffez reported on a potentially new treatment for fibromyalgia and chronic fatigue syndrome—involving neck surgery—claiming that it could be a big breakthrough for millions of people. (The segment was none-too-subtly titled "A Surgical Cure.") Those of us watching the television were more than a little skeptical about this "new treatment."

Drs. Heffez and Rosner claimed that a malformation between the upper portion of the neck and the brain stem, called a Chiari malformation (CM), could be responsible for the symptoms of fibromyalgia and chronic fatigue syndrome, along with cervical myelopathy, another cause of compression of the upper spinal cord. They said these conditions could be corrected, or certainly made better, by surgery.

Chiari malformations occur when a portion of the base of the brain protrudes into the upper spine. Small protrusions, dubbed CMI, usually don't cause symptoms and aren't found until later in life. Large protrusions (CMII), often discovered in early childhood, usually *do* trigger neurologic symptoms because they block the flow of cerebrospinal fluid.

When the natural flow of the spinal fluid is blocked by these large protrusions, the pressure damages the spinal cord, producing a cyst within it called syringomyelia. Only in very rare cases will CMI block the flow of spinal fluid. It was this more common, less serious form—Chiari malformation I, with or without syringomyelia—that was said to be a cause of fibromyalgia and chronic fatigue syndrome. And since a surgically fixable malformation was the cause, surgery was the cure.

The logic works. So far, so good.

But although people with Chiari or fibromyalgia or chronic fatigue syndrome *superficially* share symptoms of pain and functional difficulties, on closer examination, these symptoms are quite different. For example, pain in Chiari is usually confined to the neck and upper spine, whereas fibromyalgia and chronic fatigue syndrome produce pain all over the body. Psychological distress is common in fibromyalgia and chronic fatigue syndrome but not in Chiari. Those with Chiari malformation don't complain of low energy or fatigue. And neurological abnormalities are present in Chiari but not in fibromyalgia and chronic fatigue syndrome.

In addition, people with CMI are likely to suffer dysfunction of the cranial nerves. Those are the 12 nerves, originating in the skull, that govern the senses as well as other vital functions. Consequently, the disorder may impair vision, movement of the vocal cords, tongue, and facial muscles, and lead to progressive loss of balance and difficulty coordinating the feet. However, patients are *not* likely to experience difficulty concentrating, increased sensitivity to light, sound, and odors, or contend with bowel and bladder disorders—common symptoms of fibromyalgia.

Medical literature shows that CMI with active symptoms is rare, whereas fibromyalgia certainly is not (touching about 6 million to 12 million people, or 2 percent to 4 percent of the population). So if CMI does give rise to fibromyalgia, it is only in a very tiny percentage of the total number of cases.

Doctors Heffez and Rosner claimed to have performed more than 300 neck operations. According to Dr. Heffez, aside from only 8 percent of patients who did not show improvement from the surgery, "We have observed that every symptom can be improved to a greater or lesser degree." Such optimism was at odds with the surgical literature. Three large studies followed patients for two years postsurgery. Half of their neurologic symptoms did indeed improve, but 30 percent were unchanged and 20 percent were worse. Neck and shoulder symptoms were least likely to improve. A far cry from the dramatic benefits claimed by Dr. Heffez.

I addressed his reported results in an editorial in the April 2001 issue of the *Cleveland Clinic Journal of Medicine*. Not long after, Dr. Heffez responded in the same publication, "At no time in the past and at no time in the future will I prescribe any form of surgery for the treatment of fibromyalgia or the closely related disorder, chronic fatigue syndrome."

I do not feel that surgical treatment solely for fibromyalgia or chronic fatigue syndrome is a viable option. Nevertheless, as with any controversy, we all learn. I carefully screen all of my patients with either disorder for objective neurologic signs and symptoms. I prescribe appropriate testing—sometimes including an MRI scan of the brain stem and neck when a patient exhibits obvious weakness of the arms or hands, muscle wasting, abnormal or asymmetric deep tendon reflexes, severe imbalance problems after walking for a while, and/or abnormal reflexes. If these findings are prominent, I will send that patient to a neurosurgeon to be considered for appropriate surgical treatment.

Silicone Breast Implants and Chronic Fatigue Syndrome

Since the 1960s, silicone has been used both to improve the cosmetic appearance of the breast and for reconstruction after breast cancer surgery. Initial use involved direct injection of silicone gel into breast tissue, a practice especially prevalent in Japan. Later, implantation of silicone gel encased in a silicone envelope became the standard procedure. Other implants, such as a saline solution in a silicone envelope, were available, but the cosmetic effect was judged inferior.

Reports of systemic symptoms associated with silicone gel and silicone gel implants appeared sporadically in the 1960s and 1970s. Most of these reports described symptoms such as fatigue and pain in both joints and muscles. Because the symptoms were rare, nonspecific, and were also known to vex many women who'd never been exposed to silicone, they were not investigated thoroughly.

In the late 1980s and early 1990s, anecdotal reports of formally defined autoimmune diseases occurring in women with silicone breast implants began to surface. Most studied only one or a few patients. Often they came from plastic surgeons who had seen a few women with rheumatoid arthritis, lupus, scleroderma, or Sjögren's syndrome after having received silicone breast implants, and questioned whether there might be a connection. (Scleroderma is an autoimmune disease in which the skin thickens throughout the body. It can be associated with lung scarring, pulmonary artery disease, and high blood pressure with rapid kidney failure. It is in no way related to fibromyalgia.) Others reported finding positive autoantibodies, like the fairly ubiquitous, pesky, and nonspecific antinuclear antibodies (ANA) in a few implant patients. But as we learned earlier, these can occur in people without autoimmune disorders.

In the 1980s and 1990s, the estimated number of breast implant recipients was one million, and the number of reports of autoimmune disease was very small—the same small frequency that would be expected in the general population. But when the media got a whiff of the silicone breast hypothesis, it reported that many doctors were concerned about silicone breast implants. In the world of public and legal opinions, a cause and effect was established between silicone implants and autoimmune diseases.

As a result, the company that made the implants, and possibly the doctors who implanted them, faced monetary and social responsibility problems—which spurred researchers to investigate hypotheses and loosen purse strings to make such research possible. Careful studies evaluating large numbers of patients were designed and completed. They showed no association or scientific cause-and-effect relationship between silicone breast implants and autoimmune diseases.

Nonetheless, silicone implants were still under attack. Breast implant recipients were still seeking out rheumatologists in droves to determine if they had an autoimmune disease. I saw a great many of these very worried ladies, and so did other doctors. We at the Cleveland Clinic performed a study. Others observed and hypothesized too.

In one study, Dr. Gary Solomon reported in the *New England Journal of Medicine* what he considered to be a new syndrome in 176 silicone breast patients. This syndrome was characterized by fatigue (77 percent), memory problems (65 percent), diffuse joint pain (56 percent), and dry eyes (50 percent). That same year, Dr. Bruce Freundlich and colleagues described a similar syndrome in 50 breast implant recipients examined in their rheumatology practice. These patients' syndrome included fatigue (88 percent), diffuse joint pain (78 percent), joint stiffness (75 percent), and poor sleep (71 percent).

In addition, some patients had dry eyes and dry mouth. A few of these underwent biopsies of the inner lining of the mouth and were discovered to have the same inflammatory tissue structure changes under the microscope as are seen in Sjögren's syndrome. They believed that silicone gel was somehow interacting with the immune system and that this was responsible for a new autoimmune disease, which they named human adjuvant disease or silicone associated illness.

We at the Cleveland Clinic didn't think it was a new disease. In order to complete a study to prove or disprove that, however, we needed a lot of patients with symptoms and silicone breast implants to see if they were just like people who had never been exposed to silicone gel.

A large law firm contacted us, eager to send us patients with silicone breast implants and diffuse symptoms so we could characterize the symptoms and determine if they had autoimmune diseases. There was a class action lawsuit under way, and they promised to pay for the entire medical evaluations for the patients they sent us. We'd found our comparative population!

From March 1994 through September 1995, two other rheumatologists and I evaluated 76 patients with symptoms thought to be related to silicone breast implants, and 80 patients who met the diagnostic criteria for chronic fatigue syndrome. We found no differences between the groups in any signs or symptoms. Both groups exhibited the same very high frequencies of fatigue, diffuse muscle pain, and sleep disturbance (more than 84 percent in both groups). The frequency of positive autoantibodies was also the same for both groups.

We presented this information, published in abstract form at the 1995 meeting of the American College of Rheumatology, then presented a second abstract at the 1996 meeting. Our finding: there was no reason to postulate a new disease. People with silicone breast implants had stress-related symptoms. Many other similar reports reached the same conclusion.

Let's continue in a controversial vein and put fibromyalgia in societal perspective.

Chapter 7

Society, Stress, and Health

The statistics are unsettling: the United States, despite spending significant dollars on health care, is relatively unhealthy compared to most European countries. Americans have higher levels of C-reactive protein (CRP), a protein in the blood that serves as both a marker for inflammation and a measure of stress. Stress makes cells—and us—old before our time. It also robs us of deep sleep. In these many ways, CRP is linked to fibromyalgia and other chronic diseases.

The level of CRP in the blood rises as socioeconomic status falls, which fits right in with what we know about fibromyalgia: CRP rises with stress, the key player in fibromyalgia. It is also a biologic marker of inflammation and imperfect cell repair, which are important factors in increasing one's chances of developing heart and blood vessel disease.

As the middle class shrinks in the United States, the number of working poor increases, and resultant stress becomes more prevalent, is it any surprise that we are becoming unhealthier and seeing a rising number of stress-related conditions such as fibromyalgia? One interpretation is that people in the United States experience more stress than those in other countries; hence the high CRP levels.

Hold that thought.

Symptoms of Societal Stress

What kind of stress are we talking about when we say "societal stress"?

There is the serious stress that comes from being in debt, working at a job we hate, trying to be superparents (or superkids), and keeping up with the perceived pressures of a society that flaunts wealth, fashion, beauty, and possessions.

There is the constant bombardment of our senses from television, radio, iPods, cell phones, text messaging, hand-held computers, IMs, computer games, and all sorts of other technologies.

There is the stress we put on ourselves to be better, smarter, thinner, and happier.

And there is stress that others impose on us to give more of our time, or money, or selves to aging parents, those less fortunate, and our nagging consciences.

Stress is all around us, and in our fast-paced, technology-laden American society, we have little opportunity to get away from it.

Chronic societal stress has a generally negative effect on our health. We see a higher frequency of diseases that stem from inflammation and/or poor cell repair such as high blood pressure, heart disease, and diabetes, as well as an increased frequency of noninflammatory illnesses like fibromyalgia.

What about the stress ignited by a traumatic or catastrophic event? Do we see the same negative effects? Are there spikes of chronic symptoms and resulting conditions?

Let's take a look at a couple of catastrophic events and see.

Acute Stress after Catastrophic Events

Enschede, the Netherlands. On May 13, 2000, a fireworks depot exploded in a residential area of Enschede, the Netherlands. More than 900 people were injured, and 23 died. An estimated 500 homes were destroyed or damaged. The townspeople experienced sudden and catastrophic stress that impacted not only their emotions and their livelihoods but also the very fabric that made up their lives, friendships, and families.

Three weeks later, 1,567 residents who lived in the vicinity responded to a questionnaire about how they were feeling. A significant percentage—more than half in most categories—complained of fatigue; pain in their necks, shoulders, and backs; pain in their bones and muscles; as well as forgetfulness and headaches. The questionnaire didn't ask about whether the people were sleeping well, but if sleep disturbance had been a major issue too, we would have labeled the Enschede symptoms as fibromyalgia.

Taken with what we know about stress in the United States, there's little doubt: fibromyalgia symptoms are common when a population is stressed to the max.

Hurricane Andrew. When deadly Hurricane Andrew swept through southern Florida in August 1992, it left behind a swath of destroyed homes, lives, and businesses—and a pile of stress. The effect was exactly what we expected: the higher the stress caused by the traumatic event, the more fibromyalgialike symptoms were reported.

A study showed that four months after Hurricane Andrew, chronic fatigue syndrome patients in that area were in more pain than those from nearby counties. Their emotional distress was high, and they complained of fatigue, headaches, sore throats, and pain—all core symptoms of fibromyalgia and chronic fatigue syndrome.

September 11 and Terrorism. The 9/11 story is a little more complicated and a bit contradictory. Based on studies from before the terrorist attacks of September 11, 2001, we would have expected that such a huge, sudden, and immensely stressful catastrophe would produce increased fibromyalgia symptoms.

Here's what we actually learned.

Although the frequency of fibromyalgia, widespread pain, and joint and muscle pain *did* rise a little after the attack, the increase was not statistically significant. One thing did rise significantly: many women said that their pain interfered with their ability to do simple tasks of daily living after 9/11.

Just to muddle the issue, based on interviews conducted within five to eight weeks after the attack, the percentage of people with post-traumatic stress disorder and depression had risen significantly. What's more, the closer people lived to the destroyed World Trade Center, the higher the percentage.

The most common symptoms among people exposed to acute terror include headaches, back and neck pain, fatigue, sleep difficulties, digestive symptoms, and diffuse neurological symptoms. Those most vulnerable are women ages 40 to 60 with a history of anxiety, or roughly 18 percent of the general population.

Six months after 9/11, new prescriptions for antidepressant medications nearly tripled, from the national average of 8.7 percent to 21.3 percent. Three years after the 1995 Oklahoma City federal building bombing, many of the symptoms described above, much like fibromyalgia, still persisted in those at risk.

So while acute stress produces symptoms *a lot like* fibromyalgia, it may not produce "bona fide" fibromyalgia. Furthermore, different types of stress generate similar, but not necessarily exact, symptoms.

One kind of stress we've overlooked is chronic stress not induced by socioeconomic factors. A good example of this is war-related stress.

War and Chronic Stress. Let's look at stress in the 1991 Gulf War conflict as described in two pertinent articles.

In one, the data showed that ill veterans described, in order of frequency, symptoms of muscle pain and weakness, and joint, chest, and/or back pain. An average of 22 percent reported muscle symptoms, compared with 11 percent found in non–Gulf War veterans.

A couple of thoughts and observations to consider: If the muscle pain described by veterans is fibromyalgia, the frequency is much higher in *both* groups of veterans than in the general population, where it is a mere 0.5 percent for men. And why is the frequency higher in Gulf War veterans? Has the nature of war changed? Have *we* changed?

The second article was coauthored by Dr. Dennis Ang, my former colleague at the Cleveland Clinic. He and his research team identified 69 Gulf War veterans who, five years after the conflict, still had chronic widespread pain. The authors used the American College of Rheumatology criteria for fibromyalgia as the definition for widespread pain. They examined factors both prior to and during the war that differentiated the veterans who developed chronic widespread pain from those who did not. This is the perfect study for our purposes because it answers our burning question: what are the factors associated with fibromyalgia in people who find themselves in chronic stressful circumstances?

Remember, one person's stress can be another person's motivation. What we each perceive as stress is highly personal and individual. According to the researchers, the most important factors associated with chronic widespread pain were perception of stress due to military experiences at the time of the Gulf War *and* a family history of fibromyalgialike illnesses. The level of combat was a factor only if *perceived stress* was high. Of interest, neither symptoms of anxiety nor depression were associated with the chronic widespread pain, either.

For these veterans, was just being at war enough stress to cause fibromyalgia? According to Dr. Ang, "The notion that Gulf War veterans in this [study] have an increased perceptual sensitivity or altered perception to external stimuli is consistent with what has been reported by other investigators in the field."

Let's come back to that at the end of the chapter.

Stress and Alcohol Use

Dr. Ang's analysis also concluded that symptoms of alcohol use protected against chronic widespread pain. Veterans with this factor were 80 percent less likely to develop chronic widespread pain. This relationship is interesting because many contemporary studies of public health have reported that moderate alcohol use (one or two drinks a day) is protective compared to never or seldom drinking.

I'd always assumed that this was due simply to stress reduction—which may be true—but Ang and his team pointed out that there may be a relevant pain mechanism at work. As you know, people with fibromyalgia have higher than normal concentrations of the neurotransmitter NMDA in their spinal fluid. When NMDA binds to nerve receptors in the spinal cord, it sensitizes them so their response to stimulus is magnified. Alcohol can block the NMDA receptor and prevent increased sensitivity. Additionally, some researchers have observed that chronic widespread pain is significantly lower in moderate drinkers compared to those who do not drink or drink excessively.

"Everything in moderation" wins another round.

What Role Do Genes and Temperament Play?

As noted in Dr. Ang's study of Gulf War veterans, a family history of fibromyalgialike symptoms was a key factor in the development of widespread chronic pain. So why is it that a substantial portion of the general population develops FMS symptoms in the wake of a stressful episode or, more likely, with continuous major social stress? What might differentiate them from those who do not develop FMS?

One answer is genes, and another, related to genes, is temperament.

In 1993, Dr. C. Robert Cloninger, a psychiatrist and geneticist at the Washington University School of Medicine in Saint Louis, Missouri, wrote about temperament, which can be best understood as an individual's automatic emotional responses to situations in society. It's how you are hardwired to face life, and it may well be an inherited response.

Dr. Cloninger constructed a model of four dimensions of automatic emotional responses: (1) novelty seeking, (2) harm avoidance, (3) reward dependency, and (4) persistence. People who approach life with harm avoidance are cautious, organized, law abiding, and more nervous than others. Those with novelty-seeking responses are curious, disorganized, quick tempered, and impulsive. Reward-dependence traits include sensitivity and a need for societal contact. And, of course, people with the persistence trait are industrious and hardworking. He suggested that our personalities are a mixture of these traits, although with some men and women, one or another trait dominates.

Dr. Cloninger further predicted that each of these traits was attributable to different genes and closely related to brain chemistry metabolism: harm avoidance is related to serotonin pathways, novelty seeking to dopamine pathways, and the last two to norepinephrine pathways. Research since 1992 has shown that these relationships are a bit more complicated than this, but the general concept has held up.

Now it becomes interesting.

Back in chapter 3, I introduced you to the serotonin transporter gene—common in fibromyalgia sufferers—which makes people more sensitive to pain as well as to sound, bright lights, and other stimuli. Its short-allele version appears to be one of the genes central to the harm-avoidance trait. As we learned in chapter 4, this is the gene that was involved in increased fear responses, as measured by doctors at the Pittsburgh Mind-Body Center using PET scans.

This relationship between the serotonin transporter gene and the harm-avoidance trait makes sense. In the medical and psychology literature about temperament, people with harm avoidance are prone to depression, insomnia, and job dissatisfaction. They are also more likely to be creative and, according to one study, to be interpretive dancers!

In my own clinic, my fibromyalgia patients tell me that they always lock their doors, have insurance, pay their bills on time, wear their seat belts, and vote regularly. They are good, careful people—people with high harm avoidance. On the other hand, people with the long-allele version of the gene are more likely to be cigarette smokers. The long allele is not associated with harm avoidance, so they aren't very cautious.

Before we leave the discussion about genes and personality, it is important to understand that roughly 75 percent of people have genotypes with either two short alleles (25 percent) or one long allele and one short allele (50 percent). Only about 2 percent to 4 percent of the population have FMS symptoms, so being born with this gene hardly predicts the disorder in any one person. As we continue to learn more about fibromyalgia, many other genes that predispose men and women to FMS are bound to turn up. This is only one small piece of the puzzle, but an important one.

A Synthesis

What we've learned in these many chapters is that people with fibromyalgia and central sensitization have symptoms that arise from stress and disordered sleep. Why don't all people get these symptoms when they're stressed? I guess it depends on the level of stress and the individual sensitivity to stress of the people at risk.

If we consider where human beings have come from in the past 100,000 years that our species has been on Earth, we live in very special times that are very different from even the recent past. Our first attempts at literature were epic poems that celebrated heroes like Beowulf, who went off into the dark woods to slay the man-eating monster Grendel; the

Greek king Odysseus, who sailed off to great adventure. Why were these people celebrated? Because they came back. Most heroes and adventurers who entered the great woods alone or sailed beyond the sight of land never returned.

These vaunted heroes did not have high harm-avoidance traits. They were novelty seekers. The high avoidance people stayed home, procreated, planned ahead, put up stocks, and were ready for winter. They brought order and law to society. What's more, in times of societal stress, they slept lightly and gave the first alarms. In those times, they were first to hear the enemy, to perceive signs of the attacker in the woods, to smell the hunting animal's approach. It mattered little to the genes how these harm avoiders felt during times of stress. All that was important was getting through the danger safely. Anyway, most of those ancient stressful events resolved quickly and were short lived. For most of our history, having these genes was predominantly a good thing.

What of today? Is it a good thing to be a harm avoider? Not so much.

Modern technology and Thomas Edison brought us artificial lighting, so we no longer have to depend on the moon or the sun. Shift workers sleep all day and work all night, and we have unprecedented sensory input from all our technological gadgets. It's no wonder that the United States spends more than twice as much money per capita on health care than the United Kingdom, yet our citizens are less healthy.

We're all getting increasingly stressed and manifesting it as the symptoms of pain and fatigue. But who are the first people, the early warning system, who notice this state of affairs? The harm avoiders, of course, with their sensitive serotonin genes, who experience stress as symptoms. These sensitive people, whose nerves fire at lower than normal thresholds, are the canaries in our society's coal mine.

Perhaps we should heed them, because ultimately we are all at risk.

Conclusion

The main reason I wrote this book was to banish the helplessness that so often makes fibromyalgia symptoms worse. I hope I have accomplished this in several ways. One, by showing you how fibromyalgia is diagnosed. Two, by reassuring you in case you have been told otherwise that you are exhibiting a stress-related illness with a long history and a clear set of signs and symptoms. Though we can't cure fibromyalgia, doctors can treat its root causes through medication and other therapies, and you yourself can do much in the way of lifestyle changes to lessen its severity, especially by reducing stress in your life. Three, by showing you the disguises fibromyalgia assumes, such as chronic fatigue syndrome, post-traumatic stress disorder, post–Lyme disease, and others, to help you understand how to get the right diagnosis.

I wish you well in the battle against fibromyalgia. I hope that I have armed you well with the knowledge you will need to fight it—and win.

Appendix I

Helpful Resources

Support and Information Organizations

American Fibromyalgia Syndrome Association
7371 East Tanque Verde Road, Tucson, AZ 85715
(520) 733-1570
www.afsafund.org

Fibromyalgia Network
PO Box 31750, Tucson, AZ 85751-1750
(800) 853-2929
www.fmnetnews.com

National Fibromyalgia Association
2121 South Towne Centre, Suite 300, Anaheim, CA
92806
(714) 921-0150
www.fmaware.org

Major Medical Centers

Cleveland Clinic Foundation
9500 Euclid Avenue, Cleveland, OH 44195
(866) 594-2091

Health information: http://my.clevelandclinic.org/ disorders/fibromyalgia

Johns Hopkins Arthritis Center
5200 Eastern Avenue, Suite 4100, Baltimore, MD 21224
(410) 550-8089
www.hopkins-arthritis.org/arthritis-info/fibromyalgia

Mayo Clinic.com
www.mayoclinic.com/health/fibromyalgia

Finding a Physician
American College of Rheumatology
1800 Century Place, Suite 250, Atlanta, GA 30345-4300
(404) 633-3777
www.rheumatology.org
The ACR website includes a "Find a Rheumatologist" directory that's updated every two weeks.

American Medical Association
515 North State Street, Chicago, IL 60654
(800) 621-8335
www.ama-assn.org
Similarly, the AMA's website features "DoctorFinder," with information about more than 800,000 doctors and how to contact them.

Finding an Alternative Medicine Practitioner
Contact these professional organizations for the names of practitioners who are members and/or certified to practice in your state.

Acupuncture

American Academy of Medical Acupuncture (AAMA)
1970 East Grand Avenue, Suite 330, El Segundo,
  CA 90245
(310) 364-0193
www.medicalacupuncture.org

American Association of Acupuncture and Oriental
  Medicine (AAAOM)
PO Box 162340, Sacramento, CA 95816
(866) 455-7999
www.aaaomonline.org

Biofeedback

Association of Applied Psychophysiology and Biofeedback (AAPB)
10200 West 44th Avenue, Suite 304, Wheat Ridge, CO
  80033
(800) 477-8892
www.aapb.org

Hypnotherapy

American Society of Clinical Hypnosis (ASCH)
140 North Bloomingdale Road, Bloomingdale,
  IL 60108
(630) 980-4740
www.asch.net

Massage Therapy

American Massage Therapy Association (AMTA)
500 Davis Street, Suite 900, Evanston, IL 60201-4695
(877) 905-2700
www.amtamassage.org

Appendix II

The Antiquity of FMS through Pathology

In chapter 2, we saw how FMS was viewed by artists and scientists throughout history. But how have past physicians viewed it? What names have they given it? How did FMS come to be defined? One path was staked by the doctors who studied the muscles and thought the illness began there. They believed that muscle hardenings, or muscle "calluses," were the cause of the all-over pain caused by what we now call fibromyalgia.

Muscle Hardenings

The earliest interest in unexplained pain syndromes focused on anatomy and what was seen under the microscope when painful muscles were biopsied. Whether patients with muscle hardenings had what we now call FMS is an open question. Remember, we usually find only what we look for, and what we look for changes our perspective. So it was that many physicians studied the phenomenon of perceived muscle hardenings and reported varied findings.

1843: A German physician named Robert Friedrich Froriep is credited with providing the first descriptions of painful hardened areas in muscles. In 148 of 150 patients with rheumatic conditions—and without the benefit of tissue biopsies—he reported finding muscle calluses.

1908: Dr. H. Strauss identified three types of muscle calluses and, in the case of a 25-year-old named Potter, reported that surgically removing the hardened area brought relief. The pathology showed that degenerating muscle fibers were encased by connective tissue called fascia. Today we might wonder whether this was a situation caused by vascular disease and obstruction of blood flow to the muscle or the result of trauma.

1912: A German doctor by the name of A. Muller described a condition in which initial severe pain was followed by decreased pain that never completely disappeared. Usual locations were the muscles in the buttocks, between the ribs, and the abdominal muscles. Muller found pealike nodules near the breastbone and recommended massage to relieve the pain they caused. He believed that these painful muscles were "oversensitive" to pressure and theorized that symptoms worsened with psychic stress, alcohol use, or prolonged activity. However, the doctor also identified patients who had muscle pain but no nodules. This is the first historical description that sounds quite similar to what we now call fibromyalgia.

1925: Dr. F. Lange, too, biopsied, in his words, "quite a number" of muscle hardenings. He believed, but could not prove, that poor blood circulation during exercise allowed toxins to build up and create tender nodules and taut bands of painful muscle. Lange recommended a treatment called gelotripsie (GEE-lo-trip-see), which called for a blunt object to be used forcefully on all tender areas. It produced, as you might imagine, muscle tears and bruising. Not surprisingly, very few of Lange's patients returned for a second round of gelotripsie.

1932: A Dr. Ruhlman injected histamine (a local irritant produced by inflammatory cells) into the muscles of dogs, producing local inflammation. He noticed blood vessel damage at biopsy and postulated that reduced local circulation was responsible for the muscle inflammation.

1938: Czechoslovakian physician A. Reichart proposed three clinical features of painful muscles: (1) point tenderness, (2) palpable hardening, and (3) palpations that produced pain elsewhere, or referred pain. He prescribed heat massage and injecting the patient with a solution of saline or 10 percent glucose; such treatment seemed to improve symptoms.

1951: Our friend Dr. Lange performed 24 biopsies of muscle calluses; only one showed abnormalities consistent with scar tissue or inflammation. Not a very convincing defense of the muscle-callus hypothesis.

1960: Dr. K. Miehlke obtained biopsies from 77 patients. His findings led him to suggest that hypoxia (a deficiency of oxygen) due to decreased circulation and blood flow to the muscle was responsible for the pain and muscle hardenings he observed.

Less about Muscle Hardenings and More about "Fibrositis"

In his important 1904 paper, William R. Gowers attempted to describe and classify all of the musculoskeletal pain syndromes. It was a difficult task, but he accomplished it well. Among the pain syndromes that Gowers described is one he called fibrositis. He described the pain as "strictly symmetrical" and more common in the second half of life.

"The patients have been elderly ladies of blameless habits and elderly abstemious clergymen, [and] members of conspicuously gouty families." Gowers wrote, recognizing the importance of inheritance. He felt that the physiological cause was "the hypersensitivity of the muscle spindle … impulses from the muscles, which act on spinal centers, although normally these scarcely affect consciousness," which suggests nerve involvement.

"It is indeed strange," Gowers noted, "that such acute pain should be provided through structures which normally give rise to no sensation; pain due either to excessive excitation or to an induced excessive susceptibility." He recognized that the muscles of people with the disorder were more sensitive to pain than normal.

Gowers rejected the notion of the muscle callus: "There is no evidence of a hyperplastic process [scar formation]," he said. He postulated that fibrositis might be caused by inflammation but could not find evidence to prove it. He felt that hypersensitivity was caused by " … a form of inflammation of the fibrous tissue of the muscles." Unfortunately, this is probably where Gowers went wrong, unless he was referring to unexplained sensitivity of the structures.

As for treatment, Gowers touted the benefits of "free perspiration," making him one of the first advocates of aerobic exercise for the treatment of fibrositis/fibromyalgia.

1904: Scottish pathologist Dr. Ralph Stockman embraced many of Gowers's theories but felt that the pathology resulted from pressure on sensory nerves. In 1920 he studied 142 patients with symptoms of muscular stiffness, pain, and exhaustion. Stockman found only occasional nodules and normal blood tests and biopsies for these patients.

Around the same time, unfortunately, two British doctors, brothers Richard Llewellyn Jones Llewellyn and Arthur Bassett Jones published a 693-page book that essentially described all muscular, joint, bone, and "neurological pain" as fibrositis, making the term so general that it was useless.

1938: Dr. Jonas H. Kellgren, too, described referred pain when muscles were injected with a 5 percent saline solution, the same year as Czechoslovakia's Dr. Reichart was conducting his research.

1942: Dr. Janet Travell formulated the concept of the trigger point, building on Kellgren's work on referred pain, and supported the concept of local injury. This was usually treated with injections of a local anesthetic or by a technique where an aerosol anesthetic was sprayed at the site of pain. Travell published several studies. In one study of 50 patients, despite her support of a nodular theory, biopsies showed no pathological changes. In these cases, Travell hypothesized that hypoxia (low oxygen supply to the muscle due to trauma) caused the condition.

We need to be careful lest we become confused here. I had the opportunity to speak with Dr. Travell in 1978. Her definition of the trigger point differentiated it from the tender point of fibromyalgia. When a trigger point is activated by pressure, there is pain at the site of pressure with simultaneous radiation to other adjacent anatomic sites. It implies acute or chronic injury and local tissue damage that can be seen with a microscope. The tender point, by contrast, is simply an area that is hypersensitive to pressure or other stimuli, which, when activated, is painful but does not produce radiating pain. It implies a general state of hypersensitivity. To my mind, her work separated the old concepts of muscle pain from the new.

1944: Dr. Will Copeman found nodules only in areas where fat invaded holes normally used by nerves and arteries to feed and stimulate the muscle. The invasive fat eventually pinches a nerve and produces inflammation. Removing the fat or injecting it with an anesthetic improved symptoms. Copeman did not use the term *fibrositis.*

1947: Dr. Max Valentine reviewed papers about the microscopic appearance of fibromyalgia muscle biopsies and failed to find substantiating pathology with regard to muscle calluses.

As you can see, the theory of nodules causing muscle pain kept creeping back into medical theory. But even when employing the most advanced technology of the day—tissue biopsy—nodules were rarely found.

Another Pathway to FMS

If we retrace our historical steps, we might be able to clear this up. At the same time that our highly scientific pathologists were looking at muscle tissue under the microscope in an attempt to find definitive muscle pathology, a competing, more "holistic" theory was evolving.

The Greek physician and writer Galen (A.D. 129–circa 199) and his followers felt that the many symptoms experienced by individuals with diffuse pain were due to the downward flow (from the brain?) of a morbid humor (fluid) called rheuma. How can you biopsy that?

In 1869, George Beard, a neurologist of some repute, adopted this theory of rheuma and gave it a name: neurasthenia. Interestingly, the symptoms of neurasthenia included profound fatigue with fainting, disordered sleep, headaches, increased skin and muscle sensitivity, bowel problems, and diffuse spinal pain (termed by some as "spinal irritation"). This illness sounds a lot like Gowers's fibrositis and our FMS; and although proponents of neurasthenia didn't feel a need for muscle biopsy, they described "tender spots" in the majority of their patients.

Galen's theory of a central nervous system illness that produced all those symptoms was not given much credence in the medical community of his day. However, as we will see as the modern-day discussion of FMS continues, Galen was one smart guy!

Bibliography

Aaron, L. A., and D. Buckwald. "A Review of the Evidence for Overlap among Unexplained Clinical Conditions." *Annals of Internal Medicine* 134, no. 9, pt. 2 (May 1, 2001): 868–81.

Adler, G. K., and R. Geenen. "Hypothalamic-Pituitary-Adrenal and Autonomic Nervous System Functioning in Fibromyalgia." *Rheumatic Disease Clinics of North America* 31, no. 1 (February 2005): 187–202.

Aggarwal, V. R., J. McBeth, J. M. Zakrzewska, M. Lunt, and G. J. Macfarlane. "The Epidemiology of Chronic Syndromes That Are Frequently Unexplained: Do They Have Common Associated Factors?" *International Journal of Epidemiology* 35, no. 2 (April 2006): 468–76.

Anand, K. J. "Pain, Plasticity, and Premature Birth: A Prescription for Permanent Suffering?" *Nature Medicine* 6, no. 9 (September 2000): 971–73.

Ang, D. C., P. M. Peloso, R. F. Woolson, K. Kroenke, and B. N. Doebbeling. "Predictors of Incident Chronic Widespread Pain among Veterans following the First Gulf War."

Clinical Journal of Pain 22, no. 6 (July–August 2006): 554–63.

Arnold, L. M., J. I. Hudson, E. V. Hess, A. E. Ware, D. A. Fritz, M. B. Auchenbach, L. O. Starck, and P. E. Keck Jr. "Family Study of Fibromyalgia." *Arthritis and Rheumatism* 50, no. 3 (March 2004): 944–52.

Arnold, L. M., Y. Lu, L. J. Crofford, M. Wohlreich, M. J. Detke, S. Iyengar, and D. J. Goldstein. "A Double-Blind, Multicenter Trial Comparing Duloxetine with Placebo in the Treatment of Fibromyalgia Patients with or without Major Depressive Disorder." *Arthritis and Rheumatism* 50, no. 9 (September 2004): 2974–84.

Banks, J., M. Marmot, Z. Oldfield, and J. P. Smith. "Disease and Disadvantage in the United States and in England." *JAMA* 295, no. 17 (May 3, 2006): 2037–45.

Bennett, R. M. "Three Years Later: Presidential Address to Myopain "04." *Journal of Musculoskeletal Pain* 12 (2004): 1–12.

Bennett, R. "The Fibromyalgia Impact Questionnaire (FIQ): A Review of Its Development, Current Version, Operating Characteristics, and Uses." *Clinical and Experimental Rheumatology* 23, no. 5, supplement 39 (September–October 2005): S154–62.

Blumenthal, D. E. "Tired, Aching, ANA-positive: Does Your Patient Have Lupus or Fibromyalgia?" *Cleveland*

Clinic Journal of Medicine 69, no. 2 (February 2002): 143–46; 151–52.

Burckhardt, C. S. "Fibromyalgia: Novel Therapeutic Aspects." *Journal of Musculoskeletal Pain* 12, nos. 3 and 4 (2005): 65–72.

Burton, T. M. "High Hopes. Surgery on the Skull for Chronic Fatigue? Doctors Are Trying It." *Wall Street Journal*, November 11, 1999.

Buskila, D., L. Neumann, E. Zmora, M. Feldman, A. Bolotin, and J. Press. "Pain Sensitivity in Prematurely Born Adolescents." *Archives of Pediatrics and Adolescent Medicine* 157, no. 11 (November 2003): 1079–82.

Calabrese, L., T. Danao, E. Camara, and W. Wilke. "Chronic Fatigue Syndrome." *American Family Physician* 45, no. 3 (March 1992): 1205–13.

Calvo-Alén, J., H. M. Bastian, K. V. Straaton, S. L. Burgard, I. S. Mikhail, and G. S. Alarcón. "Identification of Subsets among Those Presumptively Diagnosed with, Referred, and/or Followed Up for Systemic Lupus Erythematosus at a Large Tertiary Care Center." *Arthritis and Rheumatism* 38, no. 10 (October 1995): 1475–84.

Chow H. Y., J. M. Cash, L. H. Calabrese, and W. S. Wilke. "Patients with Chronic Fatigue Syndrome (CFS) and Silicone-Associated Illness (SAI) Are Similarly Disabled." *Arthritis and Rheumatism* 39, no. 9 (supplement) (September 1996): S52.

Chow, H. Y., L. H. Calabrese, W. S. Wilke, and J. M. Cash. "Is Silicone-Associated Illness Really Chronic Fatigue Syndrome?" *Arthritis and Rheumatism* 38, no. 9 (supplement) (September 1995): S264.

Ciccone, D. S., D. K. Elliott, H. K. Chandler, S. Nayak, and K. G. Raphael. "Sexual and Physical Abuse in Women with Fibromyalgia Syndrome: A Test of the Trauma Hypothesis." *Clinical Journal of Pain* 21, no. 5 (September–October 2005): 378–86.

Clauw, D. J. "The 'Gulf War Syndrome': Implications for Rheumatologists." *Journal of Clinical Rheumatology* 4, no. 4 (August 1998): 173–74.

Clauw, D. J., R. M. Bennett, F. Petzke, M. J. Rosner, and E. Paiva. "Prevalence of Chiari Malformation and Cervical Stenosis in Fibromyalgia." *Arthritis and Rheumatism* 43 (2000) (supplement): 173.

Clauw, D. J. , P. Mease, R. H. Palmer, R. M. Gendreau, and Y. Wang. "Milnacipran for the Treatment of Fibromyalgia in Adults: A 15-Week, Multicenter, Randomized, Double-Blind, Placebo-Controlled, Multiple-Dose Clinical Trial." *Clinical Therapeutics* 30, no. 11 (November 2008): 1988–2004.

Clauw, D. J., M. Schmidt, D. Radulovic, A. Singer, P. Katz, and J. Bresette. "The Relationship between Fibromyalgia and Interstitial Cystitis." *Journal of Psychiatric Research* 31, no. 1 (January–February 1997): 125–31.

Cloninger, C. R., D. M. Svrakic, and T. R. Przybeck. "A Psychobiological Model of Temperament and Character." *Archives of General Psychiatry* 50, no. 12 (December 1993): 975–90.

Crofford, L. J., M. C. Rowbotham, P. J. Mease, I. J. Russell, R. H. Dworkin, A. E. Corbin, J. P. Young Jr., L. K. LaMoreaux, S. A. Martin, and U. Sharma. "Pregabalin for the Treatment of Fibromyalgia Syndrome: Results from a Randomized, Double-Blind, Placebo-Controlled Trial." *Arthritis and Rheumatism* 52, no. 4 (April 2005): 1264–73.

Croft, P., J. Schollum, and A. Silman. "Population Study of Tender Point Counts and Pain as Evidence of Fibromyalgia." *BMJ* 309, no. 6956 (September 17, 1994): 696–99.

Drewes, A. M., K. D. Nielsen, S. J. Taagholt, K. Bjerregård, L. Svendsen, and J. Gade. "Sleep Intensity in Fibromyalgia: Focus on the Microstructure of the Sleep Process." *British Journal of Rheumatology* 34, no. 7 (July 1995): 629–35.

Dunkl, P. R., A. G. Taylor, G. G. McConnell, A. P. Alfano, and M. R. Conaway. "Responsiveness of Fibromyalgia Clinical Outcome Measures." *Journal of Rheumatology* 27, no. 11 (November 2000): 2683–91.

Gamaldo, C. E., and C. J. Earley. "Restless Legs Syndrome: A Clinical Update." *Chest* 130, no. 5 (November 2006): 1596–1604.

Gantz, N. M., and E. E. Coldsmith. "Chronic Fatigue
Syndrome and Fibromyalgia Resources on the World Wide
Web: A Descriptive Journey." *Clinical Infectious Diseases*
32, no. 6 (March 2001): 938–48.

Gendreau, R. M., M. D. Thorn, J. F. Gendreau, J. D.
Kranzler, S. Ribeiro, R. H. Gracely, D. A. Williams,
P. J. Mease, S. A. McLean, and D. J. Clauw. "Efficacy of
Milnacipran in Patients with Fibromyalgia." *Journal of
Rheumatology* 32, no. 10 (October 2005): 1975–85.

Goldenberg, D. L. "Psychiatric and Psychological Aspects
of Fibromyalgia Syndrome." *Rheumatic Disease Clinics of
North America* 15, no. 1 (1989): 105–14.

Goldenberg, D. L., C. Burckhardt, and L. Crofford.
"Management of Fibromyalgia Syndrome." *JAMA* 292,
no. 19 (November 17, 2004): 2388–95.

Gowers, W. R. "A Lecture on Lumbago and Its Lessons."
British Medical Journal (January 16, 1904): 117–21.

Gracely, R. H., F. Petzke, J. M. Wolf, and D. J. Clauw.
"Functional Magnetic Imaging Evidence of Augmented
Pain Processing in Fibromyalgia." *Arthritis and Rheumatism*
46, no. 5 (May 2002): 1333–43.

Grann, D. "Stalking Dr. Steere over Lyme Disease."
New York Times, June 17, 2001, magazine section.

Gür, A., M. Karakoç, K. Nas, Remzi, Cevik, A. Denli,
and J. Saraç. "Cytokines and Depression in Cases with

Fibromyalgia." *Journal of Rheumatology* 29, no. 2 (February 2002): 358–61.

Hadler, N. M. "Is Fibromyalgia a Useful Diagnostic Label?" *Cleveland Clinic Journal of Medicine* 63, no. 2 (March–April 1996): 85–87.

Hariri, A. R, E. M. Drabant, K. E. Munoz, B. S. Kolachana, V. S. Mattay, M. F. Egan, and D. R. Weinberger. "A Susceptibility Gene for Affective Disorders and the Response of the Human Amygdala." *Archives of General Psychiatry* 62, no. 2 (February 2005): 146–52.

Harth, M., and W. R. Nielson. "The Fibromyalgia Tender Points: Use Them or Lose Them? A Brief Review of the Controversy." *Journal of Rheumatology* 34, no. 5 (May 2007): 914–22.

Hassett, A. L., and L. H. Sigal. "Unforeseen Consequences of Terrorism: Medically Unexplained Symptoms in a Time of Fear." *Archives of Internal Medicine* 162, no. 16 (September 9, 2002): 1809–13.

Hedenberg-Magnusson, B., M. Ernberg, and S. Kopp. "Symptoms and Signs of Temporomandibular Disorders in Patients with Fibromyalgia and Local Myalgia of the Temporomandibular System. A Comparative Study." *Acta Odontologica Scandinavica* 55, no. 6 (December 1997): 344–49.

Heffez, D. S., R. E. Ross, Y. Shade-Zeldow, K. Kostas, M. Morrissey, D. A. Elias, and A. Shepard. "Treatment of Cervical Myelopathy in Patients with the Fibromyalgia Syndrome: Outcomes and Implications." *European Spine Journal* 16, no. 9 (September 2007): 1423–33 (doi 10.1007/s00586-007-0366-2).

Held, K., H. Künzel, M. Ising, D. A. Schmid, A. Zobel, H. Murck, F. Holsboer, and A. Steiger. "Treatment with the CRH1-Receptor-Antagonist R121919 Improves Sleep-EEG in Patients with Depression." *Journal of Psychiatric Research* 38, no. 2 (March–April): 129–36.

Hellinger, W. C., T. F. Smith, R. E. Van Scoy, P. G. Spitzer, P. Forgacs, and R. S. Edison. "Chronic Fatigue Syndrome and the Diagnostic Utility of Antibody to Epstein-Barr Virus Early Antigen." *JAMA* 260, no. 7 (August 19, 1988): 971–73.

Holmes, G. P., J. E. Kaplan, J. A. Stewart, B. Hunt, P. F. Pinsky, and L. B. Schonberger. "A Cluster of Patients with a Chronic Mononucleosis-like Syndrome. Is Epstein-Barr Virus the Cause?" *JAMA* 257, no. 17 (May 1, 1987): 2297–303.

Hughes, G., C. Martinez, E. Myon, C. Taïeb, and S. Wessely. "The Impact of a Diagnosis of Fibromyalgia on Health Care Resource Use by Primary Care Patients in the UK: An Observational Study Based on Clinical Practice." *Arthritis and Rheumatism* 54, no. 1 (January 2006): 177–83.

Ismail, K., B. Everitt, N. Blatchley, L. Hull, C. Unwin, A. David, and S. Wessely. "Is There a Gulf War Syndrome?" *Lancet* 353, no. 9148 (January 16, 1999): 179–82.

Jensen, B., I. H. Wittrup, H. Røgind, B. Danneskiold-Samsøe, and H. Bliddal. "Correlation between Tender Points and the Fibromyalgia Impact Questionnaire." *Journal of Musculoskeletal Pain* 8, no. 4 (2000): 19–29.

Kales, A., C. R. Soldatos, and J. D. Kales. "Sleep Disorders: Insomnia, Sleepwalking, Night Terrors, Nightmares, and Enuresis." *Annals of Internal Medicine* 106, no. 4 (April 1987): 582–92.

Katz, R. S., F. Wolfe, and K. Michaud. "Fibromyalgia Diagnosis: A Comparison of Clinical, Survey, and American College of Rheumatology Criteria." *Arthritis and Rheumatism* 54, no. 1 (January 2006): 169–76.

Kellgren, J. H. "Observations on Referred Pain Arising from Muscle." *Clinical Science* 3 (1938): 175–90.

Kennedy, M., and D. T. Felson. "A Prospective Long-Term Study of Fibromyalgia Syndrome." *Arthritis and Rheumatism* 39, no. 4 (April 1996): 682–85.

Kroenke, K., E. E. Krebs, and M. J. Bair. "Pharmacotherapy of Chronic Pain: A Synthesis of Recommendations from Systematic Reviews." *General Hospital Psychiatry* 31, no. 3 (May 1 2009): 206–19.

Levine, P. H., P. G. Snow, B. A. Ranum, C. Paul, and M. J. Holmes. "Epidemic Neuromyasthenia and Chronic Fatigue Syndrome in West Otago, New Zealand." *Archives of Internal Medicine* 157, no. 7 (April 14, 1997): 750–54.

Lin, E. H., W. Katon, M. Von Korff, L. Tang, J. W. Williams Jr., K. Kroenke, K. Hunkeler, L. Harpole, M. Hegel, P. Arean, et al. "Effect of Improving Depression Care on Pain and Functional Outcomes among Older Adults with Arthritis: A Randomized Controlled Trial." *JAMA* 290, no. 18 (November 12, 2003): 2428–29.

Macfarlane, G. J., P. R. Croft, J. Schollum, and A. J. Silman. "Widespread Pain: Is an Improved Classification Possible?" *Journal of Rheumatology* 23, no. 9 (September 1996): 1628–32.

Marcus, D. M. "An Analytic Review of Silicone Immunology." *Arthritis and Rheumatism* 39, no. 10 (October 1996): 1619–26.

Mayhew, E., and E. Ernst. "Acupuncture for Fibromyalgia—A Systemic Review of Randomized Trials." *Rheumatology* 46, no. 5 (May 2006): 801–04 (Epub, December 19, 2006).

McWhinney, I. R., R. M. Epstein, and T. R. Freeman. "Lingua Medica: Rethinking Somatization." *Annals of Internal Medicine* 126, no. 9 (May 1, 1997): 747–50.

Mease, P. J., D. J. Clauw, L. M. Arnold, D. L. Goldenberg, J. Witter, D. A. Williams, L. S. Simon, C. V. Strand,

C. Bramson, S. Martin, et al. "Fibromyalgia Syndrome." *Journal of Rheumatology* 32 (2005): 2270–77.

Moldofsky, H., P. Scarisbrick, R. England, and H. Smythe. "Musculoskeletal Symptoms and Non-REM Sleep Disturbance in Patients with 'Fibrositis Syndrome' and Healthy Subjects." *Psychosomatic Medicine* 37 (1997): 341–51.

Nahit, E. S., I. M. Hunt, M. Lunt, G. Hunt, A. J. Silman, and G. J. Macfarlane. "Effects of Psychosocial and Individual Psychological Factors on the Onset of Musculoskeletal Pain: Common and Site-Specific Effects." *Annals of Rheumatic Diseases* 62, no. 8 (August 2003): 755–60.

Nyrén, O., L. Yin, S. Josefsson, J. K. McLaughlin, W. J. Blot, M. Engquist, L. Hakelius, J. D Boyce Jr., and H. O. Adami. "Risk of Connective Tissue Disease and Related Disorders among Women with Breast Implants: A Nationwide Retrospective Cohort Study in Sweden." *BMJ* 316, no. 7129 (February 7, 1998): 417–22.

Offenbacher, M., B. Bondy, S. de Jonge, K. Glatzeder, M. Krüger, P. Schoeps, and M. Ackenheil. "Possible Association of Fibromyalgia with a Polymorphism in the Serotonin Transporter Gene Regulatory Region." *Arthritis and Rheumatism* 42, no. 11 (November 1999): 248–88.

Paaladinesh, T., B. Alshay, M. A. Brookhart, and N. K. Choudhry. "Primary Prevention of Cardiovascular Diseases with Statin Therapy: A Meta-Analysis of Randomized

Controlled Trials." *Archives of Internal Medicine* 166, no. 21 (November 27, 2006): 2307–13.

Peterson, M. C., J. H. Holbrook, D. Von Hales, N. L. Smith, and L. V. Staker. "Contributions of the History, Physical Examination, and Laboratory Investigation in Making Medical Diagnoses." *Western Journal of Medicine* 156, no. 2 (February 1992): 163–65.

Quintner J. L., and M. L. Cohen. "Fibromyalgia Falls Foul of a Fallacy." *Lancet* 353, no. 9158 (March 27, 1999): 1092–94.

Sarac, A. J., and A. Gur. "Complementary and Alternative Medical Therapies for Fibromyalgia." *Current Pharmaceutical Design* 12, no. 1 (2006): 47–57.

Schoenfeld, P. "Efficacy of Current Drug Therapies in Irritable Bowel Syndrome: What Works and Does Not Work." *Gastroenterology Clinics of North America* 34, no. 2 (June 2005): 319–35.

Shin, L. M., S. P. Orr, M. A. Carson, S. L. Rauch, M. L. Macklin, N. B. Lasko, P. M. Peters, L. J. Metzger, D. D. Dougherty, P. A. Cannistraro, et al. "Regional Cerebral Blood Flow in the Amygdala and Medial Prefrontal Cortex During Traumatic Imagery in Male and Female Vietnam Veterans with PTSD." *Archives of General Psychiatry* 61, no. 2 (February 2004): 168–76.

Silverman, B. G., S. L. Brown, R. A. Bright, R. G. Kaczmarek, J. B. Arrowsmith-Lowe, and D. A. Kessler.

"Reported Complications of Silicone Gel Breast Implants: An Epidemiologic Review." *Annals of Internal Medicine* 124, no. 8 (April 15, 1996): 744–56.

Simons, D. G. "Muscle Pain Syndromes—Part I." *American Journal of Physical Medicine* 54, no. 6 (December 1975): 289–311.

————. "Muscle Pain Syndromes—Part II." *American Journal of Physical Medicine* 55, no. 1 (February 1976): 15–42.

Smythe, H. A. "'Fibrositis' as a Disorder of Pain Modulation." *Best Practice & Research Clinical Rheumatology* 5 (1979): 823–32.

Spitzer, R. L., K. Kroenke, J. B. W. Williams, and the Patient Health Questionnaire Primary Care Study Group. "Validation and Utility of a Self-Report Version of PRIME-MD: The PHQ Primary Care Study." *JAMA* 282, no. 18 (November 10, 1999): 1737–44.

Sridharan, S. T,. and W. S. Wilke. "Chiari Malformation and Chronic Fatigue Syndrome/Fibromyalgia: A Paradigm for Care." 1185–91. In: Benzel, E. C. *Spine Surgery: Techniques, Complication Avoidance, and Management.* 2d ed. Philadelphia: Elsevier, 2005.

Tishler, M., O. Levy, I. Maslakov, S. Bar-Chaim, and M. Amit-Vazina. "Neck Injury and Fibromyalgia—Are They Really Associated?" *Journal of Rheumatology* 33, no. 6 (June 2006): 1183–85.

Travell, J., and S. H. Rinzler. "The Myofascial Genesis of Pain." *Postgraduate Medicine* 11, no. 5 (May 1952): 425–34.

Urrows, S., G. Affleck, H. Tennen, and P. Higgins. "Unique Clinical and Psychological Correlates of Fibromyalgia Tender Points and Joint Tenderness in Rheumatoid Arthritis." *Arthritis and Rheumatism* 37, no. 10 (October 1994): 1513–20.

Van den Berg, B., L. Grievink, R. K. Stellato, C. J. Yzermans, and E. Lebret. "Symptoms and Related Functioning in a Traumatized Community." *Archives of Internal Medicine* 165, no. 20 (November 14, 2005): 2402–07.

Vitali, C., A. Tavoni, R. Neri, P. Castrogiovanni, G. Pasero, and S. Bombardieri. "Fibromyalgia Features in Patients with Primary Sjögren's Syndrome. Evidence of a Relationship with Psychological Depression." *Scandinavian Journal of Rheumatology* 18, no. 1 (1989): 21–27.

Wessely, S., C. Nimnuan, and M. Sharpe. "Functional Somatic Syndromes: One or Many?" *Lancet* 354, no. 9182 (September 11, 1999): 936–39.

White, K. P., M. Harth, M. Speechley, and T. Ostbye. "Testing an Instrument to Screen for Fibromyalgia Syndrome in General Population Studies: The London Epidemiology Study Screening Questionnaire." *Journal of Rheumatology* 26, no. 4 (April 1999): 880–84.

White, K. P., W. R. Nielson, M. Harth, T. Ostbye, and M. Speechley. "Does the Label 'Fibromyalgia' Alter Health Status, Function, and Health Service Utilization? A Prospective, Within-Group Comparison in a Community Cohort of Adults with Chronic Widespread Pain." *Arthritis and Rheumatism* 47, no. 3 (June 15, 2002): 260–65.

Wilke, W. S. "Treatment of 'Resistant' Fibromyalgia." *Rheumatic Disease Clinics of North America* 21, no. 1 (February 1995): 247–60.

———. "Fibromyalgia: More Than a Label." *Cleveland Clinic Journal of Medicine* 63, no. 2 (March–April 1996): 87–89.

———. "The Clinical Utility of Fibromyalgia." *Journal of Clinical Rheumatology* 5, no. 2 (April 1999): 97–102.

———. "Can Fibromyalgia and Chronic Fatigue Syndrome Be Cured by Surgery?" *Cleveland Clinic Journal of Medicine* 68, no. 4 (April 2001): 277–79.

———. "New Developments in the Diagnosis of Fibromyalgia Syndrome: Say Goodbye to Tender Points?" *Cleveland Clinic Journal of Medicine* 76, no. 6 (June 2009): 345–52.

Wilke, W. S., F. M. Fouad-Tarazi, J. M. Cash, and L. H. Calabrese. "The Connection between Chronic Fatigue Syndrome and Neurally Mediated Hypotension." *Cleveland Clinic Journal of Medicine* 65, no. 5 (May 1998): 261–66.

Wilke, W. S., and A. H. Mackenzie. "Proposed Pathogenesis of Fibrositis." *Cleveland Clinic Quarterly* 52, no. 2 (summer 1985): 147–54.

Wolfe, F., and K. Michaud. "Severe Rheumatoid Arthritis (RA), Worse Outcomes, Comorbid Illness, and Sociodemograghic Disadvantage Characterize RA Patients with Fibromyalgia." *Journal of Rheumatology* 31, no. 4 (April 2004): 695–700.

Wolfe, F., and J. J. Rasker. "The Symptom Intensity Scale, Fibromyalgia, and the Meaning of Fibromyalgialike Symptoms." *Journal of Rheumatology* 33, no. 11 (November 2006): 2291–99.

Wolfe, F., H. A. Smythe, M. B. Yunus, R. M. Bennett, C. Bombardier, D. L. Goldenberg, P. Tugwell, S. M. Campbell, M. Abeles, P. Clark, et al. "The American College of Rheumatology 1990 Criteria for Classification of Fibromyalgia: Report of the Multicenter Criteria Committee." *Arthritis and Rheumatism* 33, no. 2 (February 1990): 160–72.

Yunus, M., A. T. Masi, J. J. Calabro, K. A. Miller, and S. L. Feighenbaum. "Primary Fibromyalgia (Fibrositis): Clinical Study of 50 Patients with Matched Normal Controls." *Seminars in Arthritis and Rheumatism* 11 (1981): 151–71.

Zonana-Nacach, A., G. S. Alarcón, J. D. Reveille, M. Triana-Alexander, R. W. Alexander, and L. A. Bradley. "Clinical Features of ANA-Positive and ANA-Negative Patients with Fibromyalgia." *Journal of Clinical Rheumatology* 4, no. 2 (April 1998): 52–56.

Index

About the Author

William S. Wilke, MD, has worked in the Department of Rheumatic and Immunologic Diseases at Cleveland Clinic for over 35 years. He has been a member of the American College of Rheumatology, the Cleveland Rheumatism Society, the Ohio Society of Rheumatology, and the Northeastern Ohio Chapter of the Arthritis Foundation. He is previous chairman of Cleveland Clinic Pharmacy and Therapeutics Committee and a member of the *Cleveland Clinic Journal of Medicine.*

About Cleveland Clinic

Cleveland Clinic, located in Cleveland, Ohio, is a not-for-profit multispecialty academic medical center that integrates clinical and hospital care with research and education.

Cleveland Clinic was founded in 1921 by four renowned physicians with a vision of providing outstanding patient care based upon the principles of cooperation, compassion, and innovation. *U.S. News & World Report* consistently names Cleveland Clinic as one of the nation's best hospitals in its annual "America's Best Hospitals" survey. Approximately 1,800 full-time salaried physicians and researchers at Cleveland Clinic and Cleveland Clinic Florida represent more than 100 medical specialties and subspecialties. In 2007 there were 3.5 million outpatient visits to Cleveland Clinic and 50,455 hospital admissions. Patients came for treatment from every state and from more than 80 countries. Cleveland Clinic's website address is www.clevelandclinic.org.